More Advance Praise for Neurogenetics

"This really is a brilliant book which I strongly recommend. Neurogenetics can be daunting for clinicians, but the authors have produced a highly readable, up-to-date and authoritative guide. Each chapter begins with a description of an actual clinical case, and moves on to discussion of differential diagnosis and whether, when and how to proceed with genetic testing. A must for all neurologists!"

—Niall Quinn MA, MD, FRCP, FAAN, FANA
Emeritus Professor of Clinical Neurology, UCL Institute
of Neurology and Honorary Consultant Neurologist,
National Hospital for Neurology and Neurosurgery
London, England

"The field of neurogenetics seems to be advancing at light speed. Genetic causes of well-described disorders as well as newly recognized syndromes are being discovered weekly. The clinician is regularly faced with the question "What do I do now?" with little idea of where to turn. Here, Drs. Kumar, Sue, Münchau, and Klein provide a case-based, easily-digested, yet remarkably thorough and authoritative approach to lead the overwhelmed clinician out of the wilderness."

—Anthony E. Lang OC, MD, FRCPC, FAAN, FRSC, FCAHS
Lily Safra Chair in Movement Disorders, Director of the
Morton and Gloria Shulman Movement Disorders Clinic
and the Edmond J. Safra Program in Parkinson's Disease,
Toronto Western Hospital, and Jack Clark Chair in
Parkinson's Disease Research, University of Toronto
Toronto, Canada

D1446235

What Do I Do Now?

SERIES CO-EDITORS-IN-CHIEF

Lawrence C. Newman, MD
Director of the Headache Institute
Department of Neurology
St. Luke's Hospital Center
New York, NY

Morris Levin
Co-director of the Dartmouth Headache Center
Director of the Dartmouth Neurology Residency Training Program
Section of Neurology
Dartmouth Hitchcock Medical Center
Lebanon, NH

PREVIOUS VOLUMES IN THE SERIES

Pediatric Neurology
Stroke
Epilepsy
Pain
Cerebrovascular Disease
Movement Disorders

Neurogenetics

Kishore R. Kumar, MBBS, FRACP
Department of Neurogenetics
Kolling Institute of Medical Research
The University of Sydney and the Royal North Shore Hospital
St Leonards, Australia

Carolyn M. Sue, MBBS, FRACP
Department of Neurogenetics
Kolling Institute of Medical Research
The University of Sydney and the Royal North Shore Hospital
St Leonards, Australia

Alexander Münchau, Prof. Dr. Med.
Department of Paediatric and Adult Movement Disorders and
Neuropsychiatry
Institute of Neurogenetics, University of Lübeck
Lübeck, Germany

Christine Klein, MD
Institute of Neurogenetics, University of Lübeck
Lübeck, Germany

OXFORD
UNIVERSITY PRESS

Oxford University Press is a department of the University of
Oxford. It furthers the University's objective of excellence in research,
scholarship, and education by publishing worldwide.

Oxford   New York
Auckland   Cape Town   Dar es Salaam   Hong Kong   Karachi
Kuala Lumpur   Madrid   Melbourne   Mexico City   Nairobi
New Delhi   Shanghai   Taipei   Toronto

With offices in
Argentina   Austria   Brazil   Chile   Czech Republic   France   Greece
Guatemala   Hungary   Italy   Japan   Poland   Portugal   Singapore
South Korea   Switzerland   Thailand   Turkey   Ukraine   Vietnam

Oxford is a registered trademark of Oxford University Press
in the UK and certain other countries.

Published in the United States of America by
Oxford University Press
198 Madison Avenue, New York, NY 10016

Library of Congress Cataloging-in-Publication Data
Kumar, Kishore R., author.
Neurogenetics / Kishore R. Kumar, Carolyn M. Sue, Alexander Münchau, Christine Klein.
  p. ; cm.
Includes bibliographical references.
Summary: In this book, the authors use their extensive experience in the field of neurogenetics to provide
readers with a practical approach for dealing with these conditions. The 31 chapters of this book cover a broad
range of neurogenetic disorders, highlighting key issues with regards to the clinical assessment, diagnosis and
management"—Provided by publisher.
ISBN 978-0-19-938389-4 (paperback : alk. paper)
I. Sue, Carolyn M., author.   II. Münchau, Alexander, author.   III. Klein, Christine, 1969- author.
IV. Title.
[DNLM: 1. Nervous System Diseases—genetics.   2. Genetic Testing. WL 140]
RC346.4
616.8′0442—dc23
2014019689

The science of medicine is a rapidly changing field. As new research and clinical experience broaden our
knowledge, changes in treatment and drug therapy occur. The author and publisher of this work have checked
with sources believed to be reliable in their efforts to provide information that is accurate and complete, and in
accordance with the standards accepted at the time of publication. However, in light of the possibility of human
error or changes in the practice of medicine, neither the author, nor the publisher, nor any other party who has
been involved in the preparation or publication of this work warrants that the information contained herein
is in every respect accurate or complete. Readers are encouraged to confirm the information contained herein
with other reliable sources, and are strongly advised to check the product information sheet provided by the
pharmaceutical company for each drug they plan to administer.

9 8 7 6 5 4 3 2 1
Printed in the United States of America
on acid-free paper

Contents

List of Figures   xiii
List of Tables   xv
Preface   xvii
Acknowledgments   xix
Glossary of Abbreviations   xxi

1   **Early-Onset Dystonia**   1
Christine Klein
Early onset of dystonia in a limb is highly suggestive of a hereditary form of dystonia, with DYT1 dystonia being the most common form. The clinical presentation, genetic diagnosis, and treatment of early-onset dystonia is outlined in this chapter.

2   **Dopa-Responsive Dystonia**   7
Christine Klein
Dopa-responsive dystonia is typically characterized by childhood onset of dystonia, diurnal fluctuation of symptoms, and a dramatic response to levodopa therapy. In clinical practice, there is usually a considerable delay before the diagnosis of dopa-responsive dystonia is made. We will review the clinical manifestations and diagnosis of dopa-responsive dystonia, with a focus on genetic laboratory testing.

3   **Myoclonus-Dystonia**   11
Christine Klein
Myoclonus-dystonia is characterized by myoclonus and dystonia, which is action-induced, usually alcohol-responsive, and often associated with psychiatric comorbidity. Myoclonus-dystonia is caused by mutations in the *epsilon sarcoglycan* gene. We discuss how to approach patients with myoclonus-dystonia, with particular attention to genetic evaluation and family counseling.

4   **Paroxysmal Dyskinesia**   17
Alexander Münchau
Paroxysmal dyskinesias can be categorized as either paroxysmal kinesigenic dyskinesia, paroxysmal nonkinesigenic dyskinesia, or paroxysmal exertion-induced dyskinesia. Patients presenting with paroxysmal dyskinesias are often misdiagnosed as having a psychogenic (functional) disorder. The clinical phenotype, diagnosis, and treatment of these conditions is discussed in this chapter.

5 **Huntington Disease** 25

Alexander Münchau

Huntington disease is a progressive neurodegenerative disease with a devastating prognosis. The clinical phenotype is complex with a combination of abnormal movements, oculomotor abnormalities, cognitive and psychiatric symptoms. We describe the clinical phenotype and discuss how this varies according to the size of the triplet repeat in the *huntingin* gene. We also review the differential diagnosis (i.e., Huntington disease look-alikes) and the approaches to management.

6 **Dominant Parkinson Disease** 33

Christine Klein

The most common known cause of autosomal dominant Parkinson disease is mutations in the *LRRK2* gene. Other genes to consider in dominantly inherited Parkinson disease include *alpha-synuclein* and *VPS35*. The approach to patients with dominant Parkinson disease is discussed, with an emphasis on the clinical features, disease course, and treatment of Parkinson disease caused by *LRRK2* mutations.

7 **Recessive Parkinson Disease** 39

Christine Klein

Autosomal recessive Parkinson disease can be caused by mutations in the *Parkin, PINK1* and *DJ-1* genes. In this chapter, we highlight the clinical features that serve as "red flags" for recessive Parkinson disease. We discuss the indications for genetic testing and how to counsel the family.

8 **Gaucher Disease and Parkinson Disease** 45

Kishore R. Kumar and Carolyn M. Sue

Gaucher disease is caused by mutations in the *glucocerebrosidase* gene and there are a range of clinical manifestations. Furthermore, approximately 5–10% of patients with Parkinson disease have *glucocerebrosidase* mutations, making this one of the most important genetic susceptibility factors. In this chapter, the clinical manifestations of *glucocerebrosidase* mutations are discussed, with special reference to the association with Parkinson disease.

9 **Spinocerebellar Ataxia Type 2** 49

Kishore R. Kumar and Carolyn M. Sue

The causes of a spastic–ataxia phenotype are varied and include spinocerebellar ataxias (SCAs) and hereditary spastic paraplegias with signs of ataxia. Common autosomal dominant cerebellar ataxias include SCA1, SCA2, SCA3, SCA6 and SCA7. These disorders are characterized by gradual disease onset in adulthood, with progressive worsening of cerebellar and noncerebellar signs. We describe a patient presenting with adult-onset ataxia who was found to have SCA2.

10 **Spinocerebellar Ataxia Type 17** 55

Kishore R. Kumar and Carolyn M. Sue

Spinocerebellar ataxia type 17 is an autosomal dominant cerebellar ataxia with varied clinical features that include ataxia, seizures, involuntary movements (e.g. chorea and dystonia), dementia, psychiatric symptoms, corticospinal tract signs, and rigidity. In this chapter, we discuss spinocerebellar ataxia type 17, using a patient presenting with seizures and adult-onset cerebellar ataxia as an example.

11 **Sialidosis** 59

Kishore R. Kumar and Carolyn M. Sue

The clinical features of type 1 sialidosis (cherry red spot-myoclonus syndrome) include myoclonic epilepsy, visual disturbance, and ataxia in the second or third decade of life. Macular cherry red spots are always present. This condition is an autosomal recessive disorder resulting from mutations in the *NEU1* gene, and is characterized by the deficiency of α-N-acetylneuraminidase (sialidase) in leukocytes and cultured fibroblasts. We discuss the clinical manifestations and diagnosis of this condition.

12 **Friedreich Ataxia** 63

Alexander Münchau

Autosomal recessive cerebellar ataxia should be considered in patients younger than 30 years of age with a persistent and gradually worsening gait or balance disorder. Although there are many different causes, Friedreich ataxia is by far the most common. In this chapter, we summarize the clinical features, differential diagnosis, investigations, and treatment of Friedreich ataxia.

13 **Mitochondrial Encephalomyopathy, Lactic Acidosis, and Stroke-like Episodes (MELAS) Syndrome** 69

Kishore R. Kumar and Carolyn M. Sue

Important criteria for the diagnosis of MELAS syndrome include stroke-like episodes, encephalopathy, lactic acidosis, and ragged-red fibers. Most patients harbor the *m.3243A>G point mutation*. In this chapter, we use an illustrative case to underscore the cardinal clinical features of MELAS.

14 **Myoclonus Epilepsy and Ragged Red Fiber (MERRF)** 77

Alexander Münchau

In this chapter, we discuss the differential diagnosis of progressive myoclonus-ataxia epilepsy syndromes. We give particular attention to a mitochondrial encephalopathy known as myoclonus epilepsy and ragged red fibers (MERRF).

15 **POLG-Related Mitochondrial Disease** 85
Kishore R. Kumar and Carolyn M. Sue
Progressive external ophthalmoplegia is characterized by ptosis accompanied
by a progressive limitation of eye movements. Sporadic progressive external
ophthalmoplegia and sporadic Kearns-Sayre syndrome are the most common
forms, and are due to mitochondrial DNA deletions. Several nuclear-encoded
genes such as *SLC25A4, C10orf2, OPA1, TYMP,* and *POLG* can also cause
progressive external ophthalmoplegia. In this chapter we describe a patient
with progressive external ophthalmoplegia and peripheral neuropathy due to
mutations in the *POLG* gene.

16 **Mitochondrial Neurogastrointestinal Encephalopathy (MNGIE) Syndrome** 89
Kishore R. Kumar and Carolyn M. Sue
The clinical features of MNGIE (mitochondrial, neurogastrointestinal
encephalopathy) syndrome include GI dysmotility, cachexia, ptosis,
ophthalmoparesis, peripheral neuropathy, and leukoencephalopathy. MNGIE
is a rare autosomal recessive condition due to mutations in the *thymidine
phosphorylase (TYMP)* gene. We discuss the clinical features, diagnosis, and
treatment of this debilitating disease.

17 **Leber Hereditary Optic Neuropathy** 97
Kishore R. Kumar and Carolyn M. Sue
Leber hereditary optic neuropathy is characterized by bilateral (usually
sequential), painless, subacute visual loss that usually develops in early adult
life. It is caused by mutations in mitochondrial DNA and is transmitted by
maternal inheritance. In this chapter, we focus on the co-occurrence of Leber
hereditary optic neuropathy and multiple sclerosis (known as Harding disease).

18 **Charcot-Marie-Tooth Disease Type 1** 101
Alexander Münchau
Charcot-Marie-Tooth disease type 1 is characterized by a slowly progressive
motor and sensory neuropathy with foot deformities. There are several
subtypes, the most common being CMT1A caused by a 17p12 duplication
encompassing the *PMP22* gene. We describe the clinical features and discuss
how to investigate and treat this condition.

19 **Hereditary Neuropathy with Liability to Pressure Palsies** 107
Kishore R. Kumar and Carolyn M. Sue
The diagnosis of hereditary neuropathy with liability to pressure palsies
should be considered in patients with recurrent focal compressive
neuropathies and a family history consistent with autosomal dominant
inheritance. In the majority of affected individuals, there will be a 1.5-Mb
deletion at 17p11.2 that includes the *PMP22* gene. In this chapter, we discuss
the clinical features, investigations, and management of this condition.

20 **Neurofibromatosis Type 1** 113

Kishore R. Kumar and Carolyn M. Sue

The important clinical features of neurofibromatosis type 1 (von Recklinghausen disease) include café au lait patches, axillary or groin freckling, Lisch nodules in the iris, and neurofibromas. We outline the clinical manifestations, genetic diagnosis, and management of this disease.

21 **The Myotonic Dystrophies** 119

Kishore R. Kumar and Carolyn M. Sue

The myotonic dystrophies are characterized by progressive muscle degeneration leading to disabling weakness and wasting with myotonia, in combination with multisystem involvement. There are two major types of myotonic dystrophy: type 1 (also known as Steinert disease), and type 2 (also known as proximal myotonic myopathy or PROMM). In this chapter we discuss the clinical evaluation of the myotonic dystrophies with a focus on distinguishing between type 1 and type 2 disease.

22 **The Dystrophinopathies** 123

Kishore R. Kumar and Carolyn M. Sue

The dystrophinopathies include a spectrum of muscle disorders with X-linked inheritance caused by mutations in the *DMD* gene, which encodes for the dystrophin protein. Involvement of skeletal muscle can cause progressive muscle disease (Duchenne or Becker muscular dystrophy), whereas involvement of the cardiac muscle can cause DMD-associated dilated cardiomyopathy. In this chapter, the dystrophinopathies are discussed with a particular emphasis on genetic counseling and management issues.

23 **Facioscapulohumeral Dystrophy** 127

Kishore R. Kumar and Carolyn M. Sue

Facioscapulohumeral dystrophy is a common muscle disease with autosomal dominant inheritance. As the name suggests, there is a selective pattern of weakness with involvement of face, shoulder (producing scapular winging), biceps, triceps and tibialis anterior. We will review the clinical features, genetic diagnosis, and management of this disease.

24 **Inclusion Body Myopathy with Paget Disease of Bone and/or Frontotemporal Dementia** 133

Kishore R. Kumar and Carolyn M. Sue

Inclusion body myopathy with Paget disease of bone and/or frontotemporal dementia (IBMPFD) is a progressive disorder with variable penetrance chiefly affecting three main tissue types: muscle (IBM), bone (Paget disease of bone), and brain (frontotemporal dementia). It is an autosomal dominant condition caused by mutations in the *valosin-containing protein* gene. IBMPFD will be discussed in this chapter, with an emphasis on how to recognize this condition.

25 **Hereditary Spastic Paraplegia** 139
Kishore R. Kumar and Carolyn M. Sue
The term "hereditary spastic paraplegia" is applied to a group of clinically and genetically heterogenous disorders that share a primary feature, which is progressive spasticity of the lower limbs. We will discuss this condition with a focus on hereditary spastic paraplegia caused by mutations in the *SPG7* gene.

26 **Inherited Prion Diseases** 143
Alexander Münchau
Prion diseases, also referred to as transmissible spongiform encephalopathies (TSE), are caused by abnormally folded prion proteins. They occur in humans and animals, primarily affecting the central nervous system, and are invariably fatal. Prion diseases can be classified according to etiology as sporadic, acquired, or familial. In this chapter we will describe the familial forms, with particular attention to a type of prion disease known as Gerstmann-Sträussler-Scheinker syndrome.

27 **Frontotemporal Dementia—Amyotrophic Lateral Sclerosis Syndrome** 149
Kishore R. Kumar and Carolyn M. Sue
There is a close association between frontotemporal dementia (FTD) and amyotrophic lateral sclerosis (ALS) on a clinical, pathological, and genetic level. An expanded hexanucleotide repeat in the *C9ORF72* gene has recently been found to be the most common cause of familial FTD and ALS. We discuss the genetic background of FTD-ALS overlap syndromes with a focus on when to suspect that an expanded hexanucleotide repeat in the *C9ORF72* is responsible.

28 **Neurodegeneration with Brain Iron Accumulation** 155
Alexander Münchau
Neurodegeneration with brain iron accumulation (NBAI) is a large and growing group of heterogeneous disorders typically starting in childhood with variable combinations of developmental delay, dystonia, and parkinsonism. Abnormal iron deposition on MRI is a hallmark of most diseases in the NBAI spectrum with the globus pallidus and substantia nigra typically being affected. In this chapter, we review the clinical, radiological, and genetic aspects of NBAI.

29 **Coincidental Occurrence of Two Monogenic Disorders** 163
    Christine Klein
    Although the co-occurrence of mutations in more than one gene in the same patient is rare, such a finding is statistically more likely than previously thought. In this chapter, we highlight the importance of considering the co-occurrence of two neurogenetic conditions in the same patient.

30 **Direct-to-Consumer Genetic Testing** 167
    Christine Klein
    Direct-to-consumer genetic testing has enabled individuals to purchase genetic tests and receive results without the intervention of a health professional. The information provided can be difficult to interpret for the customers and their clinicians. We discuss the challenges of direct-to-consumer genetic testing in the genomics era.

31 **Incidental Findings in Genetic Testing** 171
    Christine Klein
    Given the rapid technological advances in molecular genetics, incidental findings by exome and genome sequencing or by array comparative genomic hybridization are becoming increasingly common. We discuss an approach to counseling families with regards to the detection of incidental findings on genetic testing.

Index 175

List of Figures

1-1. Pedigree of a family with DYT1 dystonia   2

2-1. Pedigree of a patient with dopa-responsive dystonia (DRD)   8

3-1. Pedigree of a family with myoclonus-dystonia   13

4-1. An example of paroxysmal kinesigenic dyskinesia with a symptomatic cause (figure from Zittel et al., with permission from Springer)   21

5-1. A girl with juvenile Huntington disease is shown   28

6-1. Pedigree of a patient with LRRK2-linked Parkinson disease   35

7-1. Pedigree of a patient with Parkin-linked Parkinson disease   41

9-1. Brain MRI (sagittal) from the patient demonstrating evidence of ponto-cerebellar atrophy   51

11-1. Fundoscopic pictures of the right (R) and left (L) eye showing bilateral cherry red spots   60

11-2. Pedigree of a family with ataxia, myoclonic epilepsy, and retinal changes   61

12-1. Typical signs of advanced Friedreich ataxia in two wheelchair-bound patients   64

13-1. Muscle biopsy from the patient with haematoxylin and eosin (H&E, panel A), nicotinamide adenine dinucleotide (NADH, panel B), succinate dehydrogenase (SDH, panel C) and modified Gomori-Trichrome (panel D) staining   71

13-2. Typical findings on brain MRI during an acute stroke-like episode in a patient with MELAS   72

14-1. Surface EMG recordings from biceps (upper trace) and triceps muscle (lower trace) are shown   78

14-2. Muscle biopsy of a patient with MERRF   80

16-1. Pedigree of family with neurological and gastrointestinal symptoms   92

16-2. Axial T2 weighted MRI in the patient showing evidence of widespread generalized increased signal intensity throughout the white matter   93

17-1. Follow-up MRI of the patient from the clinical vignette with Leber hereditary optic neuropathy   99

18-1. Ultrasound image of a median nerve section at the wrist of a patient with CMT disease type 1 (left panel) and a healthy control subject (right panel)   103

19-1. Nerve conduction studies in a patient with recurrent mononeuropathies   109

20-1. Photograph of the patient's right arm demonstrating extensive cutaneous neurofibromas   114

20-2. Photograph of the patient's eye demonstrating Lisch nodules in the iris (arrow) 116

24-1. Muscle biopsy with hematoxylin and eosin staining from the proband's brother. A rimmed vacuole is indicated by the black arrow. Adapted from a figure by Kumar et al. (2010) (with permission from Science Direct) 136

24-2. Whole-body bone scan in the patient showing evidence of widespread Paget disease of bone with involvement of the right humerus, right femur, left tibia and left hemipelvis. Adapted from a figure by Kumar et al. (2010) (with permission from Science Direct) 137

25-1. Combined cytochrome c oxidase (COX) and succinate dehydrogenase (SDH) staining of muscle tissue from the patient with a spastic-ataxia phenotype, demonstrating blue staining COX negative-SDH positive fibers 140

26-1. Relative frequency of symptoms and signs on presentation in GSS patients with P102L mutations (Webb et al., 2008) 146

27-1. Pedigree of the family with frontotemporal dementia and amyotrophic lateral sclerosis 151

28-1. MRI of the patient showing signal abnormalities in the globus pallidus (A) and substantia nigra (B) 156

28-2. MRI of a patient with pantothenate kinase-associated neurodegeneration demonstrating signal abnormalities in the globus pallidus on axial FLAIR (left panel) and coronal T2 (right panel) sequences 158

List of Tables

4-1. Classical paroxysmal dyskinesias 19

5-1. Medical treatment of chorea in adult Huntington disease patients 29

6-1. Autosomal dominant forms of Parkinson disease 36

7-1. Autosomal recessive forms of Parkinson disease 42

9-1. Results of testing for the most common genetically defined autosomal dominant cerebellar ataxias 51

10-1. Results of genetic testing for some of the autosomal dominant cerebellar ataxias 57

16-1. Nerve conduction studies in the proband suggesting a demyelinating peripheral neuropathy 91

Preface

The field of neurogenetics may prove to be quite complex and challenging for many clinicians. This is compounded by the fact that the field is developing at a rapid pace. Technological advances such as next-generation sequencing have meant that new disease-causing genes are being identified on a regular basis. It is imperative that health practitioners keep abreast of these issues and have a sound approach to dealing with these disorders.

In this book, we discuss the clinical assessment, diagnosis, molecular genetic testing, and counselling of neurogenetic conditions. The case-based format is to make the subject as clinically relevant, succinct, and engaging as possible. As authors, we have an extensive experience in the clinical and research aspects of these disorders. We bring this experience to bear by presenting a diverse range of cases that are all based on actual patients, all of whom have been seen by ourselves or our colleagues in the clinics.

We hope this book serves you well as a tool for deciphering the complexity of neurogenetic disorders.

Kishore R. Kumar, MBBS, FRACP
Department of Neurogenetics, Kolling Institute of Medical Research
and Royal North Shore Hospital, Sydney, Australia

Carolyn M. Sue, MBBS, FRACP, PhD
Department of Neurogenetics, Kolling Institute of Medical Research
and Royal North Shore Hospital, Sydney, Australia

Alexander Münchau, MD
Department of Pediatric and Adult Movement Disorders and
Neuropsychiatry, Institute of Neurogenetics, University of Lübeck,
Lübeck, Germany

Christine Klein, MD
Institute of Neurogenetics, University of Lübeck, Lübeck, Germany

Acknowledgments

DR KISHORE RAJ KUMAR

I would like to sincerely thank my wife Smitha and my daughter Ashima for their love and support. I would also like to show my appreciation to my parents, my brother Sanjeev, and my sister Kaveetha, for all their encouragement. I would also like to express my gratitude to my mother- and father-in-law, and to my sister-in-law Suma.

I would like to thank Professor Carolyn Sue and Professor Christine Klein for their supervision and mentorship. I would also like to show my gratitude to Carolyn Sue, Alexander Münchau, and Christine Klein for their help in the writing of this book. I am grateful for the support from all the laboratory staff at the Department of Neurogenetics, Kolling Institute of Medical Research, University of Sydney, and at the Institute of Neurogenetics at the University of Lübeck. I would like acknowledge the assistance of the staff from the Department of Neurology, Royal North Shore Hospital, especially Christina Liang, Kate Ahmad, Nicholas Blair, Karl Ng, Antoinette de Silva, and Fabienne Edema-Hildebrand. I am supported by the Dora Lush Postgraduate Medical Scholarship from the National Health and Medical Research Council (NHMRC) of Australia. Finally, I would to thank the patients from the neurogenetics clinic at the Royal North Shore Hospital for their invaluable cooperation.

PROFESSOR CAROLYN M. SUE

I would like to sincerely thank my husband Brett and my children Isabel and William for all their love, encouragement, and unfailing support. I am also most grateful to my parents and family for their love, dedication, and understanding. I would like to thank all my laboratory staff at the Department of Neurogenetics, Kolling Institute of Medical Research, University of Sydney, and the clinical team from the Department of Neurology, Royal North Shore Hospital, especially Christina Liang, Kate Ahmad, Nicholas Blair,

Antoinette de Silva, and Fabienne Edema-Hildebrand. I would like to also thank my mentors Cy Elliott, John G. L. Morris, Con Yiannikas, Salvatore DiMauro, and Eric Schon, as well as my patients for teaching, helping, and inspiring me to further understand disease processes that occur in neurogenetic and movement disorders. Finally, warm and whole-hearted thanks to Christine, Kishore, and Alexander for being such wonderful colleagues and friends; they have made writing this book both an educational and enjoyable task.

PROFESSOR ALEXANDER MÜNCHAU

I wish to thank my family for continuous support and patience, my patients who have taught me what I know and my mentors John P. Patten, P. Vogel, N. Quinn, K. Bhatia, M. Robertson and M. Trimble who helped me to find my way in the large world of Neurology and Neuropsychiatry. I also particularly thank C. Klein for her enormous and energetic support to set up the Department of Paediatric and Adult Movement Disorders and Neuropsychiatry in the Institute of Neurogenetics at Lübeck University. Support from the Possehl-Stiftung (Lübeck), the European Huntington Disease Network, the Deutsche Forschungsgemeinschaft and the University of Lübeck is also gratefully acknowledged.

PROFESSOR CHRISTINE KLEIN

I am most grateful to my parents, my husband Johannes, and to our children Jonas Benedikt and Hanna Felicitas for all their support, understanding, and encouragement. I would also like to express my sincere gratitude to my mentors in neurogenetics and movement disorders Xandra Breakefield, Niall Quinn, and Anthony Lang. Special appreciation is expressed to my patients for teaching and inspiring me and for generously donating time and biospecimens to help advance research in neurogenetics. A special and heartfelt thanks is extended to Carolyn Sue, Alexander Münchau, and Kishore Kumar for being such wonderful colleagues and friends and for making this book possible.

Glossary of Abbreviations

aCGH	Array comparative genomic hybridization
AD	Autosomal dominant
ADC	Apparent diffusion coefficient
ADCA	Autosomal dominant cerebellar ataxia
ALP	Alkaline phosphatase
ALS	Amyotrophic lateral sclerosis
AR	Autosomal recessive
ARSACS	Autosomal recessive ataxia of Charlevoix-Saguenay
BFIS	Benign familial infantile seizures
BHC	Benign hereditary chorea
BPAN	Beta-propeller protein-associated neurodegeneration
CJD	Creutzfeldt-Jakob disease
CK	Creatine kinase
CMT	Charcot-Marie-Tooth
CMTX	X-linked Charcot-Marie-Tooth disease
C9ORF72	Chromosome 9 open reading frame 72
COX	Cytochrome c oxidase
CSF	Cerebrospinal fluid
CT	Computerized tomography
DNA	Deoxyribonucleic acid
DRD	Dopa-responsive dystonia
DRPLA	Dentatorubral-pallidoluysian atrophy
DSD	Dejerine–Sottas disease
DTCGT	Direct-to-consumer genetic testing
ECG	Electrocardiogram
EEG	Electroencephalography
EMG	Electromyography
EPM2A	Epilepsy, progressive myoclonic type 2A
EOPD	Early onset Parkinson disease
FA	Friedreich ataxia
FAHN	Fatty acid hydroxylase-associated neurodegeneration
FLAIR	Fluid attenuated inversion recovery

FSHD	Facioscapulohumeral dystrophy
FTD	Frontotemporal dementia
GBA	Glucocerebrosidase
GCHI	GTP-cyclohydrolase I
GI	Gastrointestinal
GLUT1	Glucose transporter type 1
GPi	Globus pallidus internus
GSS	Gerstmann-Sträussler-Scheinker
HD	Huntington disease
HDL1	Huntington disease-like 1
HMSN	Hereditary motor and sensory neuropathy
HNPP	Hereditary neuropathy with liability to pressure palsies
HSP	Hereditary spastic paraplegia
HSV	Herpes simplex virus
IBMPFD	Inclusion body myopathy with Paget disease of bone and/or frontotemporal dementia
ICCA	Infantile convulsions and choreoathetosis
INAD	Infantile neuroaxonal dystrophy
iPD	Idiopathic Parkinson disease
LHON	Leber hereditary optic neuropathy
MD	Myoclonus-dystonia
MECP2	Methyl-CpG-binding-protein 2
MELAS	Mitochondrial encephalomyopathy, lactic acidosis, and stroke-like episodes
MERRF	Myoclonus epilepsy with ragged red fibers
MLPA	Multiplex ligation-dependent probe amplification
MNGIE	Mitochondrial, neurogastrointestinal encephalopathy
MoCA	Montreal Cognitive Assessment
MPAN	Mitochondrial membrane protein-associated neurodegeneration
MRI	Magnetic resonance imaging
MRS	Magnetic resonance spectroscopy
MS	Multiple sclerosis
m/s	Meters per second
mtDNA	Mitochondrial deoxyribonucleic acid
NBIA	Neurodegeneration with brain iron accumulation

NF1	Neurofibromatosis type 1
PAS	Periodic acid–Schiff
PCR	Polymerase chain reaction
PD	Parkinson disease
PED	Paroxysmal exertion-induced dyskinesia
PEG	Percutaneous gastrostomy
PEO	Progressive external ophthalmoplegia
PKAN	Pantothenate kinase-associated neurodegeneration
PKD	Paroxysmal kinesigenic dyskinesia
PNKD	Paroxysmal non-kinesigenic dyskinesias
PRNP	Prion protein (gene symbol)
PROMM	Proximal myotonic myopathy
PrP	Prion protein
PRRT2	Proline-rich transmembrane protein 2
qPCR	Quantitative polymerase chain reaction
SCA	Spinocerebellar ataxia
SDH	Succinate dehydrogenase
SENDA	Static encephalopathy with neurodegeneration in adulthood
SEP	Somatosensory evoked potential
SGCE	Epsilon sarcoglycan
SNAP	Sensory nerve action potential
SSPE	Subacute sclerosing panencephalitis
TDP-43	TAR DNA binding protein-43
TH	Tyrosine Hydroxylase
TOR1A	TorsinA
TPN	Total parenteral nutrition
TYMP	Thymidine phosphorylase
UPDRS	Unified Parkinson's Disease Rating Scale
VCP	Valosin-containing protein
VEP	Visually evoked potential
VIM	Ventral intermediate
VOR	Vestibular ocular reflex
WBBS	Whole body bone scan

Neurogenetics

1   Early-Onset Dystonia

You are asked to see a 7-year-old girl who has been referred for assessment of involuntary twisting and tremulous movements of her right hand and reduced right-hand dexterity. The girl is right-handed but has recently switched to her left hand for writing and other fine motor tasks. These symptoms have been present for about one year, are slowly progressive, and first became apparent when she started learning to write at the age of six years. Her father reports that he has been suffering from mild problems with writing since his early twenties and that the girl's brother has been diagnosed with dystonia at the age of 9 years. In the brother, the dystonia progressed relatively rapidly to involve all four extremities and the trunk and is now generalized at age 10 years. The family is worried that the condition may be familial and that the girl may be developing a similar clinical picture as her brother.

On examination, the girl shows dystonic movements of her right hand and arm that are accompanied by a dystonic tremor when she is writing or drawing a spiral. At rest, the dystonia is very mild and is exacerbated by certain postures, such as stretching out her arms in front of her, or by fine motor tasks of the right hand. There is also very mild dystonic posturing of the left hand. The remainder of the neurological examination is entirely normal. Examination of the accompanying father reveals mild right-sided writer's cramp, which is entirely task-specific. The father brought a video of his son, which shows severe generalized dystonia sparing only the face and neck.

What do you do now?

HOW DO YOU ESTABLISH A DIAGNOSIS OF DYT1 DYSTONIA?

DYT1 dystonia, also known as Oppenheim dystonia (Klein and Fahn, 2013), is a hereditary form of isolated dystonia that is caused by a mutation in the *TorsinA* (*Tor1A*) gene. In the isolated dystonias, dystonia is the only clinical feature, which may or may not be accompanied by dystonic tremor. Early onset of dystonia in a limb is highly suggestive of a hereditary form of dystonia with DYT1 dystonia being the most common.

If the neurological examination is otherwise unremarkable, complex forms of dystonia (formerly referred to as "secondary dystonia") are unlikely. Dystonic muscle contractions causing posturing of a foot, leg, or arm are the most common presenting features. Dystonia is usually first noted when performing specific actions, such as writing or walking. Over time, the dystonic movements frequently, but not invariably, occur with less specific actions, may be present at rest, and spread to other body regions (Raymond and Bressman, 1993). In our index patient, the dystonia initially developed only when writing, was later present with almost any motor task of the hands or arms, and spread to involve the contralateral arm. Unlike in her brother, the dystonia was, however, not apparent when she was at rest. In contrast, the father's dystonia remained entirely task specific and presented as pure writer's cramp (Figure 1-1).

Given the absence of any neurological signs other than dystonia/dystonic tremor and the positive family history, a genetic test may even be considered the first-line diagnostic investigation, which may precede other (expensive and/or invasive) diagnostic tests, such as a brain magnetic resonance

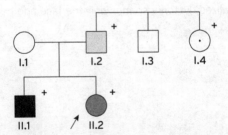

FIGURE 1-1 Pedigree of a family with DYT1 dystonia. Males are represented by squares, females by circles. The index patient is indicated with an arrow. Filled symbols mark affected individuals. Different shades of gray/black correspond to disease severity (black: generalized dystonia; dark gray: bibrachial dystonia; light gray: right-sided writer's cramp). The dot symbolizes a nonmanifesting carrier. The plus sign indicates presence of the GAG deletion in the *Tor1A* gene.

imaging (MRI) or a lumbar puncture. Notably, in DYT1 dystonia, as well as in other isolated dystonias, all ancillary investigations are normal.

Other hereditary forms of isolated dystonia include DYT6 dystonia, which is caused by mutations in the *THAP1* gene (Fuchs et al., 2009). DYT6 dystonia tends to start in adolescence and predominantly affects the upper body half, commonly with severe involvement of the face and neck and spasmodic dysphonia, whereas DYT1 dystonia usually spares the cranio-cervical region. A recently identified form of adult-onset, isolated dystonia (DYT25) is due to mutations in the *GNAL* gene (Fuchs et al., 2009). Similarly to *THAP1* mutations, *GNAL* mutations are predominantly associated with dystonia in the upper body half, which usually remains segmental. To date, only two patients have been reported with a childhood onset, making *GNAL* mutations an unlikely differential diagnosis. Finally, patients with dopa-responsive dystonia caused by mutations in the *GCH1* gene may present in childhood with isolated dystonia, usually of the legs. Dopa-responsive dystonia (DRD) may be associated with features of parkinsonism, although parkinsonism tends to develop much later than the dystonia, which may precede the parkinsonism by decades. Furthermore, DRD is characterized by a striking response to treatment with levodopa, which is not observed in DYT1 dystonia. However, any child with limb-onset dystonia should undergo a levodopa trial.

Genetic testing for DYT1 dystonia is recommended in any patient with isolated dystonia and an age of onset below 26 years (Bressman et al., 2000). This single criterion is 100% sensitive, with specificities of 63% in patients of Ashkenazi Jewish extraction to 43% in non-Jewish patients. Due to a genetic founder effect, DYT1 dystonia is considerably more common in the Ashkenazi Jewish population. Testing patients with an onset after age 26 years may be warranted in those having an affected relative with early-onset dystonia (Bressman et al., 2000).

DYT1 dystonia is one of the rare examples of a hereditary disease that is caused by a single, recurrent mutation, regardless of the ethnicity of the patient. A three-base pair (GAG) deletion in the *Tor1A* gene is the only known, confirmed cause of DYT1 dystonia. A small number of additional mutations in this gene have been reported, however, their pathogenicity has not yet been convincingly established. Therefore, a specific genetic test for the GAG deletion in *Tor1A* can be considered sufficient when trying to establish a diagnosis of DYT1 dystonia. This genetic test is commercially widely available and inexpensive. In patients with a typical early-onset generalized isolated torsion dystonia with onset in a limb, about 72% will carry the GAG deletion in the *DYT1* gene (Klein et al., 1999).

HOW DO YOU COUNSEL THE FAMILY?

DYT1 dystonia is inherited in an autosomal dominant fashion with reduced penetrance and variable expressivity. This observation is also illustrated by our DYT1 family, given that the father' sister (I.4) is entirely unaffected despite carrying the mutation, a phenomenon known as reduced penetrance. In DYT1 dystonia, penetrance is reduced to 30%, that is, only three out of ten mutation carriers are expected to develop signs of dystonia. In our family, penetrance is higher, with three out of four mutation carriers being affected. However, of the former, only one patient (II.1) suffers from severe dystonia, whereas the father (I.2) is very mildly affected. In fact, if it had not been for our index patient (II.2) who recently developed dystonia, the positive family history in this pedigree may not even have been recognized, since neither the family nor the family doctor or child neurologist had previously considered a shared cause of the father's mild writer's cramp and his son's severe childhood-onset generalized dystonia. Thus, when establishing a family history, it is imperative to keep in mind the phenomena of reduced penetrance and variable expressivity. Importantly, it is currently almost impossible to predict whether a mutation carrier will become affected and, if so, to what degree. As a general rule, patients with an earlier age of onset tend to have more severe disease with a higher likelihood of generalization. Conversely, if a mutation carrier has not developed any symptoms or signs by age 26 years, there is a good chance that he/she will remain unaffected throughout his/her life.

HOW DO YOU TREAT DYT1 DYSTONIA?

Oral medications should be tried first, including anticholinergics such as trihexiphenidyl. Although these medications are usually only moderately effective (for less than half the patients), they are sometimes helpful and usually well tolerated in high doses, such as 20 mg of trihexiphenidyl three times a day. However, cognitive side effects including inattention and poor concentration should be monitored closely, particularly in schoolchildren. Other options include baclofen and antiepileptic medications, again usually with a moderate effect at best. Botulinum toxin injections into dystonic muscles may be helpful especially for focal symptoms. Deep brain stimulation of the globus pallidus internus has been proven to be an effective treatment option including for children (Raymond & Bressman, 1993). There is currently no causative or disease-modifying treatment.

KEY POINTS TO REMEMBER ABOUT EARLY-ONSET DYSTONIA

- DYT1 dystonia is always caused by the same GAG deletion in the *DYT1* gene, making genetic testing easy and inexpensive.
- Genetic testing of the *Tor1A* gene should be considered in any patient with isolated dystonia beginning before the age of 26 years, or in a patient with later onset isolated dystonia of a limb *and* a positive family history.
- Although DYT1 dystonia follows an autosomal dominant inheritance pattern, penetrance (likelihood of developing the disease in a mutation carrier) is markedly reduced and the clinical spectrum is very broad, ranging from mild writer's cramp to severe generalized dystonia (variable expressivity).
- Disease manifestation and the clinical course cannot be predicted in an individual mutation carrier/patient; however, an early age of onset is associated with a higher tendency of the dystonia to generalize, whereas dystonia rarely manifests in mutation carriers beyond the age of 26 years.

Further Reading

Bressman, S. B., Sabatti, C., Raymond, D., de Leon, D., Klein, C., Kramer, P. L.,... Risch, N. J. (2000). The DYT1 phenotype and guidelines for diagnostic testing. *Neurology*, 54(9), 1746–1752.

Fuchs, T., Gavarini, S., Saunders-Pullman, R., Raymond, D., Ehrlich, M. E., Bressman, S. B., & Ozelius, L. J. (2009). Mutations in the THAP1 gene are responsible for DYT6 primary torsion dystonia. *Nature Genetics*, 41(3), 286–288.

Klein, C., & Fahn, S. (2013). Translation of Oppenheim's 1911 paper on dystonia. *Movement Disorders, 28*(7), 851–862.

Klein, C., Friedman, J., Bressman, S., Vieregge, P., Brin, M. F., Pramstaller, P. P.,...Sims, K. B. (1999). Genetic testing for early-onset torsion dystonia (DYT1): introduction of a simple screening method, experiences from testing of a large patient cohort, and ethical aspects. *Genet Test, 3*(4), 323–328.

Raymond, D., & Bressman, S. B. (1993). Early-onset primary dystonia (DYT1). In R. A. Pagon, M. P. Adam, T. D. Bird et al. (Eds.)., *GeneReviews.* Seattle, WA: University of Washington.

2 Dopa-Responsive Dystonia

A 13-year-old girl is referred to your neurogenetics clinic with a suspected clinical diagnosis of dopa-responsive dystonia (DRD). She developed involuntary inward turning of her right foot at the age of 8 years, which was initially only present upon exercise such as walking long distances. A year later, the dystonic movement spread to involve the left foot and leg but remained more pronounced after physical exercise. Although there was usually no dystonia in the morning, signs were more pronounced in the afternoon and evening, resulting in a bizarre dystonic gait. Due to the unusual clinical presentation, the patient was initially diagnosed with a "functional disorder." At the age of 12 years, the girl was referred to a neuropediatrician who considered a diagnosis of dopa-responsive dystonia and conducted a levodopa trial. The response to levodopa was excellent, resulting in almost complete remission of the dystonia 30 minutes after administration of the drug. The girl is now treated with a regular dose of 50 mg of levodopa three times a day and continues to enjoy a very good treatment response.

On examination during the "on" state (on levodopa treatment), you observe mild dystonic posturing of the arms and a slight postural tremor of both hands. The remainder of the motor and general neurological examination is unremarkable.

The patient's father was said to possibly have had some "movement problems," but he died in a motor vehicle accident when the patient was a small child. Both of his siblings were reportedly healthy. In addition, one of the father's maternal uncles had developed Parkinson disease (PD) at the age of 58 years (Figure 2-1).

Although a diagnosis of DRD seemed highly likely, the patient and her mother requested genetic testing in order to confirm an organic disorder. Molecular testing of the *GTP-cyclohydrolase I* (*GCHI*) gene was performed and reported to be normal.

What do you do now?

iven the typical clinical presentation and the exquisite response to levodopa, you do not doubt a diagnosis of DRD. You first ask the patient for the genetic testing report to find out exactly what kind of molecular analysis has been performed. It turns out that the genetic testing laboratory has carried out a sequence analysis of all coding exons of the *GCHI* gene and of the exon-intron boundaries. However, no quantitative (gene dosage) analysis was performed to test for deletions or duplications of whole exons. You contact the laboratory with a request for multiplex ligation-dependent probe amplification (MLPA) of the patient's DNA. MLPA is a quantitative analysis to detect possible gene dosage changes and revealed a heterozygous deletion of the entire *GCHI* gene, which was undetectable by sequence analysis. As for many other genes causing neurogenetic disorders, gene dosage changes are an important type of mutation in the *GCHI* gene, accounting for about 20% of all patients with clinically typical DRD (Hagenah et al., 2005).

The patient's grandmother (I.3), an asymptomatic family member, did not want to undergo genetic testing. However, the same heterozygous deletion of the *GCHI* gene was confirmed in her brother (I.1) who is affected with PD. Thus, it is highly likely that both the paternal grandmother (I.3) and the patient's deceased father (II.2) carried the familial mutation.

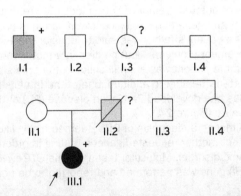

FIGURE 2-1 Pedigree of a patient with dopa-responsive dystonia (DRD). Males are represented by squares, females by circles. A diagonal line through the symbol indicates a deceased individual. The index patient is marked with an arrow. The black symbol indicates DRD, light gray symbolizes unspecified "movement problems" and dark gray Parkinson disease. The plus sign indicates a confirmed heterozygous deletion of the entire *GCHI* gene. The question marks indicate unknown mutational status (in this case, these individuals are presumed to carry the mutation).

Although the grandmother is an example of reduced penetrance of the *GCHI* mutation; the father's "movement problems" may possibly have been related to the mutation (Figure 2-1).

DRD is typically characterized by childhood onset of dystonia, diurnal fluctuation of symptoms, and a dramatic response to levodopa therapy. Later in the course of the disease, parkinsonian features may occur and may, in rare cases, be the only sign of the condition, as in individual I.1 in the present DRD family.

GCHI mutation carriers show a high degree of both inter- and intrafamilial phenotypic variability and reduced penetrance. Although penetrance is lower among men compared to women, the underlying mechanisms affecting penetrance are not yet resolved. Although the *GCHI* gene was the first gene to be discovered for a monogenic form of dystonia almost 20 years ago, there is still a considerable diagnostic delay of about 13 years on average (Tadic et al., 2012). Of further note, many mutation carriers display some residual (dystonic and/or parkinsonian) features, as also seen in our patient who had mild dystonic posturing and tremor.

To date, more than 100 different mutations, spread across the entire *GCH1* coding region, have been reported and include missense, nonsense, and splice-site mutations, small and large (whole-exon or whole-gene) deletions, and mutations in the untranslated regions.

There are also rare autosomal recessive forms of DRD, which are caused by mutations in other genes encoding proteins involved in dopamine synthesis. Of these, *Tyrosine Hydroxylase* (*TH*) gene mutations are the most common. Importantly, mutations in *TH* cause a much more severe clinical phenotype than *GCH1* mutations and resemble the phenotype observed in the rare carriers of homozygous *GCH1* mutations (Brüggemann et al., 2012).

HOW DO YOU COUNSEL THE FAMILY?

You reassure the girl and her mother that she does indeed suffer from inherited, molecularly confirmed DRD. The risk to any future offspring of the girl to inherit the mutation is 50%. As penetrance is markedly reduced, the risk to develop DRD for any future mutation carrier is less than 100% but cannot be predicted in an individual case. You also tell the family that DRD usually remains exquisitely responsive to levodopa treatment throughout the patient's life, and that medication side effects (such as dyskinesias) are very rare. You continue to follow the patient in clinic and closely monitor her treatment response, as small adjustments of the dose may become necessary over time with increasing weight and/or hormonal changes, given that the therapeutic window of the levodopa dose is usually rather small.

KEY POINTS TO REMEMBER ABOUT DOPA-RESPONSIVE DYSTONIA

- The most common cause of Dopa-responsive dystonia (DRD) are dominantly inherited mutations in the *GTP-Cyclohydrolase I (GCHI)* gene.
- The mutational spectrum of *GCHI* is broad and includes heterozygous deletions of whole exons or of the entire gene, which are not detectable by conventional sequencing and require gene dosage analysis.
- Likewise, *GCHI* mutations are associated with a wide phenotypic spectrum ranging from no symptoms or signs (reduced penetrance) to full-blown DRD or late-onset Parkinson disease.
- Although DRD was the first genetic form of dystonia to be discovered and is exquisitely treatable, there is still an average diagnostic delay of 13 years.

Further Reading

Brüggemann, N., Spiegler, J., Hellenbroich, Y., Opladen, T., Schneider, S. A., Stephani, U.,... & Klein, C. (2012). Beneficial prenatal levodopa therapy in autosomal recessive guanosine triphosphate cyclohydrolase 1 deficiency. *Archives of Neurology*, 69(8), 1071–1075.

Hagenah, J., Saunders-Pullman, R., Hedrich, K., Kabakci, K., Habermann, K., Wiegers, K.,... & Klein, C. (2005). High mutation rate in dopa-responsive dystonia: detection with comprehensive GCHI screening. *Neurology*, 64(5), 908–911.

Tadic, V., Kasten, M., Bruggemann, N., Stiller, S., Hagenah, J., & Klein, C. (2012). Dopa-responsive dystonia revisited: Diagnostic delay, residual signs, and nonmotor signs. *Archives of Neurology*, Sep 17, 1–5.

3 Myoclonus-Dystonia

You assess a 25-year-old carpet layer who has been suffering
from a movement disorder since early childhood, the cause of
which so far remains unknown. In kindergarten he was noted
to be a clumsy child who would frequently drop objects. His
mother reported that he had always had problems eating with a
spoon or drinking from a glass. Furthermore, almost any motor
task was accompanied by sudden jerky movements involving the
upper half of the body and the neck. These jerks were initially
infrequent but had become invariably present with any voluntary
motor task. Beginning in the third grade, the patient developed
a right-sided writer's cramp, as well as involuntary posturing of
his neck. His medical history was further remarkable for severe
joint problems resulting in bilateral knee and unilateral hip
replacements in his early 20s. In addition, the patient reported
several depressive episodes and a period of alcohol addiction
from his late teens to early 20s. The patient experiences a
dramatic alleviating effect on the jerks and postures when
ingesting alcohol. However, he has abstained from alcohol in
the past two years in order to avoid episodes of drunkenness
interfering with his work, and because he was found to have
abnormally elevated liver enzymes. There were no other affected
members in the family.

At rest, moderate latero- and torticollis was present, as well
as mild truncal dystonia. When stretching out his arms, the
patient developed dystonic posturing of both arms and hands,
accompanied by irregular myoclonic jerks of the shoulders and
neck. The patient also had marked writer's cramp. Pouring
water from one cup into another was impossible because of
severe action-induced myoclonus. Gait was normal, as was the
remainder of the neurological examination.

What do you do now?

HOW DO YOU ESTABLISH A DIAGNOSIS
OF MYOCLONUS-DYSTONIA?

Myoclonus-dystonia (M-D) is a hereditary movement disorder, which often starts in early childhood. The only known genetic cause of M-D is mutations in the *epsilon sarcoglycan* (*SGCE*) gene. It is not uncommon that M-D first manifests at the age of two or three years as "clumsiness" when trying to grab and hold objects. Myoclonic jerks are action-induced, further interfering with fine finger and hand movements. As M-D may be mild and not obvious at rest, it is important to provoke the myoclonic (and dystonic) movements in such cases, for example, by asking the patient to pour water from one cup into another.

Sometimes, action-induced myoclonus is mistaken for intention tremor. However, M-D is not associated with any cerebellar signs. Conversely, patients with writer's cramp and dystonic tremor or with tremulous cervical dystonia are sometimes erroneously suspected to have M-D. Importantly, unlike dystonic tremor, the "jerky movements" (i.e., myoclonus) in M-D are not necessarily present in the same muscle group or even body region. Typically, an M-D patient with writer's cramp will develop myoclonic jerks in the shoulder and neck. M-D is usually more pronounced in the upper body half; the gait may be entirely normal. Most patients develop a combination of myoclonus and dystonia; however, a small subset of patients may present with isolated myoclonus or, rarely, with isolated dystonia (Klein and Munchau, 2013).

As illustrated by our patient, there are several additional clinical features that may serve as "red flags" for M-D and improve diagnostic accuracy (Carecchio et al., 2013). For example, a broad spectrum of psychiatric features has been reported in mutation carriers, most commonly anxiety (60%), followed by depression (30%) (Weissbach et al., 2013), obsessive-compulsive disorder, and alcoholism (Peall et al., 2013). However, it remains a matter of debate whether alcoholism is an integral part of the spectrum of psychiatric comorbidity or merely the result of "self-medication."

Similar to our case, a subset of M-D patients manifest unusual (non) neurological signs that are seemingly unrelated to the movement disorder. It is important to note any such signs because they may be caused by the same underlying *SGCE* mutation, that is, a deletion of the *SGCE* affecting neighboring genes and thus causing additional phenotypes (Grunewald et al., 2008). Commonly, these deletions involve the *COL1A2* gene, resulting in skeletal features, or more rarely, the *KRIT1* gene, leading to cavernous cerebral malformations (Asmus et al., 2007).

Of further note, penetrance of the autosomal dominantly inherited *SGCE* mutations is markedly reduced (not every mutation carrier manifests the disease), which may even lead to apparently sporadic occurrence of M-D, like in our patient. The *SGCE* gene is maternally imprinted (Muller et al., 2002) leading to a seemingly paternal pattern of inheritance of M-D, such that the majority of mutation carriers who have inherited the mutated allele from their father will develop the disease, whereas those who have inherited the mutation from their mother will (almost always) remain unaffected throughout their lives (Figure 3-1).

Given the typical history and clinical findings of alcohol-responsive, action-induced myoclonus-dystonia with depression, and knowledge about the markedly reduced penetrance due to maternal imprinting of *SGCE*, genetic testing for *SGCE* mutations is indicated even in the absence of a positive family history.

Most other conditions in which myoclonus is a prominent feature are accompanied by a variety of neurological symptoms and signs that usually

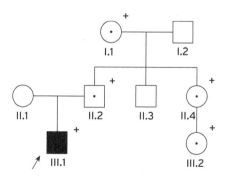

FIGURE 3-1 Pedigree of a family with myoclonus-dystonia. Males are represented by squares, females by circles. The index patient is indicated with an arrow. The filled symbol marks the only affected family member. The dots symbolize non-manifesting carriers, the plus sign indicates the presence of a deletion in the SGCE (and the neighboring COL1A2) gene. Due to maternal imprinting/paternal expression of SGCE, III.1 is the only manifesting carrier, as he inherited the mutation from his father.

are not associated with M-D and thus not mistaken for M-D. Genetic disorders with myoclonus as a major component include Unverricht-Lundborg disease, progressive myoclonus epilepsy of the Lafora type, myoclonus epilepsy with ragged red fibers (MERRF), sialidosis, neuronal ceroid lipofuscinosis and dentatorubral-pallidoluysian atrophy (DRPLA). Furthermore, benign hereditary chorea (BHC) may somewhat resemble M-D. However, in contrast to the action-induced myoclonus of M-D, jerks in BHC do not increase with complex motor tasks (Raymond and Ozelius, 1993).

Genetic testing for *SGCE* mutations is recommended in any patient with suspected M-D. Importantly, comprehensive mutational screening includes both qualitative (DNA sequencing) and quantitative (gene dosage) testing. The latter is usually carried out by multiplex ligation-dependent analysis (MLPA), which is able to identify deletions of entire exons or heterozygous deletions of the whole *SGCE* gene, an important type of mutation in M-D. When the entire *SGCE* gene is deleted, neighboring genes are commonly also involved in the deletion and, ideally, the breakpoints of the deletion should be determined. While sequencing and MLPA of the *SGCE* gene are widely available commercially, breakpoint analysis is usually performed on a research basis in collaboration with a laboratory focusing on M-D research.

HOW DO YOU COUNSEL THE FAMILY?

Myoclonus-dystonia is inherited in an autosomal dominant fashion, although there is markedly reduced penetrance due to maternal imprinting of the *SGCE* gene. As seen in the family of this patient, he is the only member apparently affected by M-D. All of the other mutation carriers (I.1, II.2, II.4, and III.2) inherited the mutation from their mothers, that is, the imprinted allele, which is thus not expressed. However, when counseling an M-D patient or *SGCE* mutation carrier, it is important to point out that the risk to pass on the mutated allele to their offspring will remain 50%, as in any dominant disease.

M-D usually starts very early in life and tends to remain relatively stable until puberty. In puberty, further disease progression is frequently noted, which then plateaus in the late teens or early 20s with no further decline. Rarely (<10%), patient may experience a spontaneous amelioration of symptoms in adult life.

Parents of children with M-D, as well as adult M-D patients, should be warned about the risk of alcoholism. Furthermore, counseling should include the increased prevalence of various psychiatric disorders associated with M-D.

Finally, if atypical signs are present, such as skeletal or cartilaginous abnormalities or brain malformation, one should suspect a contiguous gene syndrome due to a deletion of not only *SGCE* but also neighboring genes.

HOW DO YOU TREAT MYOCLONUS-DYSTONIA?

Oral medications should be tried first, such as anticholinergics, antiepileptics, and benzodiazepines. The latter may be very helpful in improving the myoclonus but may lead to addiction. Several case reports have described a moderate to good response to high doses of levodopa (500–1000 mg in adults) (Raymond and Ozelius, 1993). Some patients benefit from local botulinum toxin injections into muscles particularly affected by the dystonia and/or myoclonus.

Deep brain stimulation of the globus pallidus internus (GPi) or ventral intermediate (VIM) nucleus of the thalamus seem to be a very effective treatment for myoclonus-dystonia with GPi stimulation achieving even

---

KEY POINTS TO REMEMBER ABOUT MYOCLONUS-DYSTONIA

- Myoclonus-dystonia (M-D) is characterized by action-induced, usually alcohol-responsive myoclonus and dystonia, often associated with psychiatric comorbidity.
- Genetic testing for *SGCE* mutations should include both sequencing and gene dosage analysis, as deletions of individual exons or the entire *SGCE* gene are an important type of mutation.
- Although following an autosomal dominant inheritance pattern, penetrance (likelihood of developing the disease in a mutation carrier) is markedly reduced due to maternal imprinting of the *SGCE* gene.
- This means that family members inheriting the mutation from their mother will most likely never manifest disease; conversely, when the mutation is inherited through the father, the mutation carrier is highly likely to develop M-D.

greater improvement on the dystonia than VIM stimulation (Rughani and Lozano, 2013).

Further Reading

Asmus, F., Hjermind, L. E., Dupont, E., Wagenstaller, J., Haberlandt, E., Munz, M.,...& Gasser, T. (2007). Genomic deletion size at the epsilon-sarcoglycan locus determines the clinical phenotype. *Brain*, *130*(Pt 10), 2736–2745.

Carecchio, M., Magliozzi, M., Copetti, M., Ferraris, A., Bernardini, L., Bonetti, M.,...& Valente, E. M. (2013). Defining the epsilon-sarcoglycan (SGCE) gene phenotypic signature in myoclonus-dystonia: a reappraisal of genetic testing criteria. *Movment Disorders*, *28*(6), 787–794.

Grunewald, A., Djarmati, A., Lohmann-Hedrich, K.,Farrell, K., Zeller, J.A., Allert, N.,...& Klein, C. (2008). Myoclonus-dystonia: significance of large SGCE deletions. *Human Mutation*, *29*(2), 331–332.

Klein, C., & Munchau, A. (2013). Progressive dystonia. *Handbook of Clinical Neurology*, *113*, 1889–1897.

Muller, B., Hedrich, K., Kock, N., Dragasevic, N., Svetel, M., Garrels, J.,...& Klein, C. (2002). Evidence that paternal expression of the epsilon-sarcoglycan gene accounts for reduced penetrance in myoclonus-dystonia. *American Journal of Human Genetics*, *71*(6), 1303–1311.

Peall, K. J., Smith, D. J., Kurian, M. A., Wardle, M., Waite, A.J., Hedderly, T.,...& Morris, H. R. (2013). SGCE mutations cause psychiatric disorders: clinical and genetic characterization. *Brain*, *136*(Pt 1), 294–303.

Raymond, D., & Ozelius, L. (1993). Myoclonus-dystonia. In R. A. Pagon, M. P. Adam, T. D. Bird, C. R. Dolan, C. T. Fong, and K. Stephens (Eds.), *GeneReviews*. Seattle, WA.

Rughani, Al., & Lozano, A. M. (2013). Surgical treatment of myoclonus dystonia syndrome. *Movement Disorders*, *28*(3), 282–287.

Weissbach, A., Kasten, M., Grunewald, A., Bruggemann, N., Trillenberg, P., Klein, C., & Hagenah, J. (2013). Prominent psychiatric comorbidity in the dominantly inherited movement disorder myoclonus-dystonia. *Parkinsonism Related Disorders*, *19*(4), 422–425.

4 Paroxysmal Dyskinesia

A 14-year-old boy presents to the neurology outpatient department accompanied by his mother. She reports that for the last two years or so he has had odd "attacks" that involve writhing of the body, flinging of the arms, and arm jerking. Because they predominantly occur when he attempts to run, they have been interpreted as pertaining to disobedience and puberty revolt against school sports. His parents perceive him as a sporty character and had planned to send him to a special sports school. Other doctors and school teachers had advised psychological support. A psychiatrist suggested psychotherapy because he suspected a deep inner conflict between becoming independent and being loyal toward the parents, causing a conversion disorder.

During history taking it becomes clear that he has up to 50 attacks per day, triggered by sudden movements or rapid muscle contractions. They last less than a minute and are typically preceded by a brief premonitory sensation akin to tingling, mainly in the trunk. Immediately after an attack there is a brief period when further attacks do not occur. He has never lost consciousness or fallen during an attack. His past medical history is unremarkable. There is no family history of note. The neurological examination is normal and an assessment of his mental state is also unremarkable.

What do you do now?

To better understand the nature of these attacks, you need to see them. Unfortunately, a video of an attack is not available. You ask the patient to come to the hospital corridor, give the command "Ready, Set, Go!", and let him run.

A few seconds after starting to run the patient suddenly develops dystonic posturing of the right arm lasting for a few seconds followed by bilateral ballistic arm movements, neck extension, body twisting and dystonic gait, which lasts for less than 20 seconds and then gradually subsides. The patient remains fully conscious, can keep his balance, but appears distressed. After the attack his neurological examination is normal.

His mother confirms that you have witnessed a typical attack. Given the onset age, precipitating factors and attack phenomenology, a diagnosis of paroxysmal kinesigenic dyskinesia (PKD) can be made.

PKD belongs to the group of paroxysmal dyskinesias that are characterized by attacks of chorea, athetosis, ballism, or dystonia triggered by defined stimuli. These attacks can be symptomatic, for example, they can be caused by inflammatory lesions in the basal ganglia or thalamus (see Figure 4-1), but are mainly genetic in origin. They are typically classified into three types: PKD, induced by sudden movements or muscle contractions, as in this case; the paroxysmal nonkinesigenic dyskinesias (PNKD) triggered by alcohol, coffee, or stress; and paroxysmal exertion-induced dyskinesia (PED) caused by longer-lasting (20 minutes or more) voluntary muscle activity (Table 4-1).

Attacks in patients with PKD, the most common paroxysmal movement disorder, typically last from 10 seconds up to 5 minutes. Interictally, affected patients have no neurological signs. PKD usually starts during childhood or early adulthood, responds very well to antiepileptic drugs including carbamazepine, phenytoin, or lamotrigine, and has an excellent prognosis. Most cases are sporadic, but about a third show an autosomal dominant mode of inheritance. Most familial and many nonfamilial cases are caused by mutations in the *proline-rich transmembrane protein 2* (*PRRT2*) gene, located on chromosome 16p11.2. Interestingly, these mutations also underlie the syndrome of benign familial infantile seizures (BFIS). BFIS is characterized by clusters of complex-partial and generalized tonic-clonic seizures in the first months of life with a benign outcome, that is, normal psychomotor development and rare seizures in adulthood. Some individuals with *PRRT2* gene mutations are affected by both attacks of PKD and BFIS. In families with

TABLE 4-1 **Classical paroxysmal dyskinesias**

	Main features	Gene mutation	Inheritance	Treatment
PKD	*Attack duration:* seconds up to 5 minutes *Frequency:* up to 100/day *Triggers:* rapid movements or muscle contractions	*PRRT2*-gene Allelic conditions: – ICCA-syndrome – BFIS – rare cases of hemiplegic migraine, episodic ataxia, and paroxysmal torticollis	Autosomal dominant, incomplete penetrance	Excellent response to most anticonvulsants including carbamazepine, phenytoin, and lamotrigine
PNKD	*Attack duration:* 10 minutes up to many hours *Frequency:* Several per week or less *Triggers:* alcohol, coffee, stress	*PNKD*-gene Another gene locus on chromosome 2q31	Autosomal dominant, high penetrance	Difficult; some response to benzodiazepines, acetazolamide, gabapentin, or anticholinergic drugs
PED	*Attack duration:* 5 to 120 minutes *Frequency:* variable, depending on degree of exercise. *Trigger:* exertion for 20 minutes or more	SLC2A1-gene	Autosomal dominant, incomplete penetrance	Ketogenic diet; occasionally responding to anticonvulsants

BFIS, benign familial infantile seizures; ICCA, infantile convulsions and choreoathetosis; PED, paroxysmal exertion-induced dyskinesia; PKD, paroxysmal kinesigenic dyskinesia; PNKD, paroxysmal non-kinesigenic dyskinesia; *PRRT2*, proline-rich transmembrane protein 2; *SLC2A1*, glucose transporter 1.

these mutations, some affected family members may have PKD attacks, others BFIS, and some a combination of both, a situation that has been referred to as infantile convulsions and choreoathetosis (ICCA) syndrome.

PNKD is most often familial with a high penetrance and is caused by mutations in the *PNKD* gene (formerly known as the *MR1* gene). In most cases with PED there are mutations in the *SLC2A1* gene encoding the glucose transporter type 1 (Glut1) of the blood-brain barrier.

Paroxysmal dyskinesias, in particular PKD, can be confused with psychogenic (functional) disorders. The term *psychogenic* is much debated, and insight into the underlying mechanisms of these common and diverse disorders is limited. Considering psychological mechanisms in suddenly occurring abnormal movements is important in view of a good prognosis when adequate psychological treatment is initiated. "Psychogenic" is best considered a working hypothesis until more accurate diagnoses including a somatization or conversion disorder can be made. But when should such a working hypothesis be formulated? When the clinical presentation is unusual, that is, deviating from expected or well-established phenomenology of "organic" brain disease? In this circumstance, the term "unusual" is ambiguous and very much depends on the experience and subspecialization of the clinician using it. PKD is a good example of this dilemma. It is uncommon, odd, and can resemble some bizarre attacks of conversion disorder. However, clearly it is not a psychological disorder. It follows a distinct pattern in terms of onset, evolution, and semiology differing from patterns in patients with somatization or conversion disorder. And, importantly, patients with the latter have symptoms and signs that set them apart from other disorders including nonanatomical sensory disturbance, give-way weakness, agonist-antagonist co-contraction without dystonic posturing, distractibility and entrainment of extra movements by external rhythms to name but a few. None of these signs are present in PKD patients. This is to say that great caution should be taken to label disorders that are unknown, "unusual," or difficult to understand as "psychogenic," which is often the case in patients with paroxysmal movement disorders.

Should additional tests be carried out in our 14-year-old patient? Since he has had attacks for two years without any neurological sign in between attacks, further investigations including brain imaging, neurophysiology or screening for metabolic disorders are not mandatory. The treatment response will confirm the diagnosis.

He was put on a low dose of Carbamazepine (200 mg mane), which led to an immediate remission. He now only has occasional premonitory sensations but no further attacks of extra movements.

Genetic confirmation of the diagnosis can be considered. Testing for *PRRT2* gene mutations is now available in most diagnostic testing laboratories, and is sometimes offered as a panel covering all three classical forms of paroxysmal dyskinesias.

Additional investigations should be ordered though in patients where paroxysmal attacks start later in life (beyond the age of 20), have atypical features or are accompanied by interictal neurological abnormalities, e.g. mild pyramidal signs or abnormal joint position sense, because brain lesions can cause attacks mimicking PKD (see Figure 4-1).

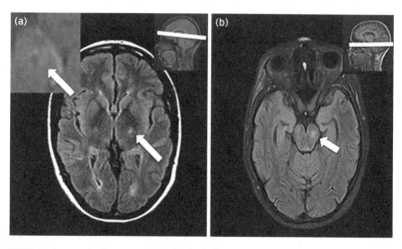

FIGURE 4-1 An example of paroxysmal kinesigenic dyskinesia with a symptomatic cause (figure from Zittel et al., with permission from Springer). A 34-year-old previously healthy woman presented with a two-week history of episodes of right-sided numbness, tingling, and spasms of her hand and leg occurring 2-15 times a day for 60 seconds. Episodes were triggered by sudden movements, such as after turning her head, or moving in bed. Neurological examination at rest was unremarkable. When running on the spot or hyperventilating, right-sided paroxysmal choreoathetosis developed and disappeared within 60 seconds. Given the patient's age and unusual features (numbness and tingling during the attack, hyperventilation as a trigger), brain imaging was performed. (a) A cerebral MRI showed an inflammatory lesion in the left lateral thalamus (fluid-attenuated inverse recovery image; arrows mark responsible lesions). Upper left panel: Gd-enhancement. Upper right panel: inset topogram shows level of axial sections. Additionally, 10 supratentorial, sub- and juxtacortical T2 lesions were observed [an example of a brainstem lesion is shown in (b)]. Cerebrospinal fluid analysis showed oligoclonal bands. A diagnosis of multiple sclerosis was made. Steroids led to prompt remission of episodes within a few days.

The prognosis of PKD is very good. The condition is treatable. Even without treatment attacks tend to occur less frequently and are less severe as patients get older.

KEY POINTS TO REMEMBER ABOUT PAROXYSMAL DYSKINESIAS

- Paroxysmal kinesigenic dyskinesia (PKD) is characterized by brief attacks of a mixed movement disorder triggered by sudden movements or muscle contractions, which can occur up to 100 times a day.
- Due to the unusual, sometimes bizarre presentation, it is often confused with a psychogenic (functional) disorder.
- Most PKD cases are sporadic but about a third are caused by autosomal dominant *PRRT2* gene mutations that also underlie BFIS.
- Structural brain lesions, predominantly in the basal ganglia and thalamus, can cause attacks resembling PKD.
- Treatment with anticonvulsants is very effective and the prognosis of PKD is excellent.

Further Reading

Becker, F., Schubert, J., Striano, P., Anttonen, A. K., Liukkonen, E., Gaily, E.,...& Weber, Y. G. (2013). PRRT2-related disorders: further PKD and ICCA cases and review of the literature. *Journal of Neurology, 260*, 1234–1244.

Demirkiran, M., & Jankovic, J. (1995). Paroxysmal dyskinesias: clinical features and classification. *Annals of Neurology, 38*, 571–579.

Kertesz, A. (1967). Paroxysmal kinesigenic choreoathetosis. *Neurology 17*, 680–690.

Mink, J. W. (2007). Paroxysmal dyskinesias. *Current Opinions in Pediatrics, 19*, 652–656.

van Vliet, R., Breedveld, G., de Rijk-van Andel, J., Brilstra, E., Verbeek, N., Verschuuren-Bemelmans, C.,...& Kievit, A. (2012). PRRT2 phenotypes and penetrance of paroxysmal kinesigenic dyskinesia and infantile convulsions. *Neurology, 79*, 777–784.

Wang, J. L., Cao, L., Li, X. H., Hu, Z. M., Li J. D., Zhang, J. G.,...& Tang, B. S. (2011). Identification of PRRT2 as the causative gene of paroxysmal kinesigenic dyskinesias. *Brain, 134*, 3490–3498.

Weber, Y. G., Storch, A., Wuttke, T. V. Brockmann, K., Kempfle, J., Maljevic, S.,...& Lerche, H. (2008). GLUT1 mutations are a cause of paroxysmal exertion-induced dyskinesias and induce hemolytic anemia by a cation leak. *Journal of Clinical Investigations*, *118*, 2157–2168.

Zittel, S., Bester, M., Gerloff, C., Münchau, A., & Leypoldt, F. (2012). Symptomatic paroxysmal kinesigenic choreoathetosis as primary manifestation of multiple sclerosis. *Journal of Neurology*, *259*, 557–558.

5   Huntington Disease

A 12-year-old girl is referred to the neuropediatric department for assessment of her dystonia. Her mother accompanies her and reports that she developed intermittent involuntary head turning and twisting around the age of 7 years. At the time, this was interpreted as "benign paroxysmal torticollis of childhood." However, the abnormal head and neck postures became continuous over a period of one year. Also, she developed bilateral arm posturing during various activities and had increasing difficulties with writing. At the age of 10 years she started to walk more slowly with inversion of both feet. Some relatives had commented on spontaneous facial grimacing. She was assessed elsewhere and given a tentative diagnosis of "primary segmental dystonia." Of late, her speech has become slightly slurred and she was noted to have difficulty with concentration at school. There is no past medical history of note. In terms of the family history, her mother has separated from her biological father years ago because of alcohol abuse and intolerable impulsivity. She is no longer in contact with the child's father or his family.

On examination, the girl is shy and somewhat slow but interacting with you in a friendly way. Her cognition and behavior appear poorly developed for her age and sometimes she has difficulties following the conversation. The horizontal eye movements are marginally slow and gaze fixation is impersistent. Bulk and strength of muscles are normal. There is generalized dystonia with facial and lingual involvement in addition to cervical, bi-brachial and bilateral leg dystonia. Also, there is some axial involvement. The dystonia is present at rest but is more pronounced during action. Her finger movements are slow over and above dystonia and there is mild rigidity in both arms. Tendon reflexes are brisk bilaterally; Babinski sign is negative. Coordination is slow but otherwise normal. Her gait is slow and dystonic with slight impairment of postural reflexes. Her speech is slow and dysarthric.

What do you do now?

The cardinal feature in this case is dystonia. The most relevant decision to be taken by the assessing physician is whether it is isolated dystonia or not. For patients with isolated dystonia, the clinical symptoms can be severe and progressive but are usually not life threatening and often manageable in a satisfactory way, as is the case, for instance, with DYT-TOR1A early-onset generalized dystonia (DYT1). However, in the case under discussion, there are signs that argue against an isolated dystonia syndrome. First, neck-onset would not be very typical in children with isolated dystonia, whereas leg or arm onset is much more common. Furthermore, involvement of facial muscles and dystonia present at rest point toward a complex form of dystonia. Finally, there are additional neurological signs including slow eye movements, speech abnormalities, mild arm rigidity, and possible cognitive impairment.

The list of possible causes of complex dystonias is long, so that comprehensive inpatient evaluation is often necessary. However, even thorough investigations cannot compensate for the lack of important historical information. Obviously, the crucial question is whether there is a relevant family history of medical illness. Therefore, great care should be taken to acquire a detailed family history.

In a separate interview, the mother volunteers that her former husband's father developed neurological symptoms in his 60s. He became demented, and was observed to be very fidgety, restless, and frail by the age of 70 years. She described her husband as impulsive and argumentative and found his social behaviour intolerable. In later years he also developed "jerky" movements, became withdrawn and started neglecting his personal hygiene. She had suspected some sort of family affliction but this was never formally assessed.

With this background of presumed autosomal dominant inheritance, and possible anticipation with a variable age-dependent clinical presentation (with hyperkinetic movements predominating in adult-onset cases and dystonia and parkinsonian features in childhood- or adolescent-onset cases), the differential diagnosis is narrowed and Huntington disease (HD) becomes the most likely diagnosis.

HD has a prevalence of at least 3–7 in 100,000 and typically presents between the age of 35 and 45 years. It is a complex neuropsychiatric disorder with an age-dependent combination of movement disorders (generalized dystonia and parkinsonism in children; generalized chorea in the early stages of adult disease with later development of dystonia, parkinsonism, and cerebellar signs), oculomotor abnormalities including gaze impersistence, early problems with antisaccades and later slowing and restriction of eye movements in all planes, and a plethora of behavioural and psychiatric symptoms. The latter include apathy, depression, impulse regulation problems, withdrawal, frontal executive disturbances in early stages, and impaired memory function, visuo-constructive deficits, apraxia, and aphasia later in the course of the disease. Other common manifestations include repetitive behaviors resembling obsessive-compulsive disorder, perseveration, and thought disorder that can lead to frank psychosis. As the disease progresses, all previously acquired cognitive and social functions are gradually lost to leave the family with a completely dependent, often difficult-to-manage patient. Also, swallowing difficulties and weight loss are typical in advanced disease. The mean survival is 15 to 18 years.

Genetics of Huntington Disease

HD is caused by an extended CAG repeat in the coding sequence of the *huntingtin* gene on the short arm of chromosome 4. Near the 5′- terminal of this gene, the CAG triplet is repeated 5–26 times in healthy controls. Individuals with triplet repeats between 27 and 35 ("intermediate alleles") are not at risk for the disease. However, due to instability of these alleles, their offspring may have disease-causing repeat expansions. Individuals with 36–39 repeats have a low risk to develop HD. Larger repeat expansions will inevitably lead to HD, provided the patient lives long enough. These expansions are unstable, that is, the number of repeats will often increase in the following generation, which explains anticipation in future generations because repeat length is inversely related to onset age.

Given the girl's clinical presentation and family background, genetic testing for HD was carried out, confirming the diagnosis of HD. The repeat size was 84, which explains the early age at onset. CAG repeat increases are larger and age at onset in affected children earlier in paternal transmission, as in this case.

Juvenile HD, also referred to as the "Westphal variant," affects about 10% of patients and is dominated by dystonia and parkinsonism but not

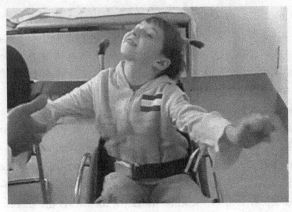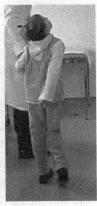

FIGURE 5–1. A girl with juvenile Huntington disease is shown. There is marked generalized dystonia affecting the face, arms and legs, trunk and neck with prominent retrocollis.

chorea. Psychomotor regression, cognitive and behavioral problems occur early in the disease course. Cerebellar signs, myoclonus, tics, and seizures can be also part of the clinical spectrum. Due to the larger repeat size, children can manifest symptoms before their parents (Figure 5-1).

Differential Diagnosis

Of the patients with an HD phenotype and autosomal dominant inheritance, most will have HD. In the remaining fraction of patients the following HD lookalikes have to be considered: (a) autosomal dominant Huntington disease-like 1 (HDL1) caused by *prion protein* gene mutations; (b) autosomal dominant HDL2 caused by mutations in the *junctophilin-3* gene; (c) HDL3, which has only been described in a few families and follows autosomal recessive inheritance; (d) autosomal dominant spinocerebellar ataxia (SCA) 17, also referred to as HDL4, and SCA 1 and 3; (e) Friedreich ataxia; (f) autosomal dominant dentatorubral-pallidoluysian atrophy and a number of disorders belonging to the group of "neurodegeneration with brain iron accumulation (NBAI)" syndromes, including autosomal dominant neuroferritinopathy and autosomal recessive pantothenate kinase-associated neurodegeneration (PKAN). Of late, it has been shown that about 2% of HD lookalike patients have repeat expansions in the *C9orf72* gene.

Management

So far no disease-modifying or neuroprotective agents are available. Treatment is symptomatic and supportive. Patients and families benefit a lot when looked after in specialized interdisciplinary HD centers that are often part of larger HD networks including the European Huntington Network. These centers offer genetic counseling; psychosocial support; medical and surgical treatment; and help to arrange physiotherapy, speech, and language therapy with the help of local general practitioners.

General measures including a high caloric diet, family and social support are often more important than medical treatment.

Chorea is typically treated with dopamine blocking agents (see Table 5-1). It has to be emphasized though that treatment should be tailored to the needs of patients and not their relatives (or the treating physician). Often, patients are hardly bothered by hyperkinetic movements and are much more impaired by social withdrawal, apathy, and depression. As treatment for depression, sulpiride can be useful because it also has an antichoreatic effect. However, serotonin reuptake inhibitors are the treatment

TABLE 5-1 **Medical treatment of chorea in adult Huntington's disease patients**

Agent	Starting daily dosage Frequency x dosage (mg)	Usual maintenance daily dosage Frequency x dosage (mg)	Evidence	Recommendation
Tiapride	3 x 50	3 x 100 to 3 x 200	↑	A
Tetrabenazine	1–2 x 12.5	50–100 (total daily dose)	↑↑	A
Sulpiride	3 x 50	3 x 100 to 3 x 200	↑	B
Olanzapine	1 x 5	1 x 10 to 1 x 15	↔	B
Haloperidol	2–3 x 1	3 x 2 to 3 x 5	↔	C
Pimozide	1 x 2	1 x 4 to 1 x 6	↔	C
Aripiprazole	1 x 2.5	1 x 5 to 1 x 15	↔	C

Evidence and recommendation according to evidence-based medicine rules; ↑↑ = randomized controlled trials or systematic meta-analyses available supporting usefulness; ↑ = nonrandomised controlled trials or case control trials available; ↔ = case series or cohort studies available; A = should be offered when indicated; B = should be considered; C = may be considered.

of choice. Anticholinergic drugs are less favorable given their risk to further exacerbate cognitive problems. Impulsivity is a common problem and can be alleviated by treatment with fluoxetine, sertraline or olanzapine. Anxiety and insomnia can be treated with mirtazapine and zoldipem. Overt psychosis should first be treated with olanzapine with quetiapine as an alternative.

KEY POINTS TO REMEMBER ABOUT HUNTINGTON DISEASE

- Huntington disease (HD) is a complex autosomal dominant neuropsychiatric disease with a variable age-dependent clinical presentation and a devastating prognosis.
- It is caused by an extended CAG-repeat in the coding sequence of the *huntingtin* gene on chromosome 4.
- Individuals with 36–39 repeats are at a low risk of developing the disease, whereas those with repeat sizes of 40 or larger will become symptomatic.
- A small fraction of patients with an HD phenotype and autosomal dominant inheritance will have conditions other than HD (HD look-alikes) including disorders belonging to the NBIA family.
- Patients and relatives should be treated in specialized interdisciplinary HD centres offering genetic counselling, psychosocial support, medical and surgical treatment and coordination of physiotherapy, speech and language therapy and other local services.

Further Reading

Bates, G., Harper, P., & Jones, L. (2002). *Huntington's disease.* New York, NY: Oxford University Press.

Bruyn, G. W., & Went, C. N. (1986).Huntington's chorea. In P. J. Vinken, G. W. Bruyn, & H. L. Klawans (Eds.), Handbook of clinical neurology (pp. 267–314). Amsterdam, Netherlands: North Holland.

Mestre, T., Ferreira, J., Coelho, M. M., Rosa, M., & Sampaio, C. (2009). Therapeutic interventions for symptomatic treatment in Huntington's disease. *Cochrane Database Systematic Review*, CD006456.

Ross, C. A., & Tabrizi, S. J. (2001). Huntington's disease: From molecular pathogenesis to clinical treatment. *Lancet Neurology, 10*, 83–98.

Tabrizi, S. J., Scahill, R. I., Durr, A., Roos, R. A. C., Leavitt, B. R., Jones R.,...& Stout, J. C. (2011). Biological and clinical changes in premanifest and early stage Huntington's disease in the TRACK-HD study: The 12-month longitudinal analysis. *Lancet Neurology, 10*, 31–42.

Wild, E. J., & Tabrizi, S. J. (2007). Huntington's disease phenocopy syndromes. *Current Opinions in Neurology, 20*, 681–687.

6   Dominant Parkinson Disease

You assess a 66-year-old retired truck driver who was diagnosed with Parkinson disease (PD) at the age of 62 years. In retrospect, he had first noticed an intermittent resting tremor and increasing clumsiness of his right hand when working on his miniature train set at around 60 years of age. The patient's symptoms and signs are well controlled with a medium dose of a long-acting dopamine agonist and rasagiline. The patient is referred to you by his attending neurologist because of a concern that the patient's PD might be familial. His brother developed PD at the age of 58 years and his mother had suffered from both PD and dementia at an advanced age. The patient has two children aged 35 and 39 years, respectively, and five grandchildren. Although none of his children or grandchildren complain of any symptoms suggestive of PD, the patient anxiously seeks genetic testing because he fears that he may have passed on the disease to his offspring. He is accompanied by both of his children when he comes to your office.

On examination, the patient has a mild right-sided resting tremor and mild bilateral bradykinesia of hand movements, more pronounced on the right-hand side. There was slight rigidity in the right arm but no postural instability. Gait was normal, apart from reduced arm swing on the right. The patient scored 12/108 points on the motor part of the Unified Parkinson's Disease Rating Scale (UPDRS III) and 27/30 points on the Montreal Cognitive Assessment (MoCA). The remainder of the neurological examination was unremarkable. Examination of the accompanying children was also entirely normal.

What do you do now?

HOW DO YOU ESTABLISH A DIAGNOSIS OF DOMINANT PARKINSON DISEASE?

The patient's family history with both an affected brother and mother is suggestive of a dominantly inherited form of PD. There are currently three well-established forms of dominant PD with mutations in the *LRRK2* gene being by far the most common known cause (Singleton et al., 2013). Although a number of different mutations in this gene have been found to be pathogenic, most patients with LRRK2-linked PD carry the same p.G2019S missense mutation. In some populations, such as Ashkenazi Jews and North African Arabs, this is due to a founder effect and explains the very high prevalence of LRRK2-linked PD of up to 30–40% of PD patients in these populations. However, the p.G2019S mutation has also arisen independently and is recurrently present in all studied populations. The frequency of this particular mutation is 4% in patients with hereditary PD of mixed ethnic background and accounts for 1% of all cases with sporadic PD (Healy et al., 2008). As in our case, the age at onset is comparable to that of idiopathic PD (iPD), as are all the clinical features (note that the term *classical* PD is sometimes considered preferable to *idiopathic* PD since it refers to a phenotype most people associate with PD without making a statement on etiology). There is, however, evidence that both motor and nonmotor signs may be more benign in LRRK2-linked disease than in iPD (Healy et al., 2008). Penetrance of *LRRK2* mutations is reduced and age-dependent. However, cases of octogenarians who remain entirely unaffected despite the presence of a pathogenic *LRRK2* mutation have been described.

According to the recommendations for genetic testing of PD patients from the European Federation of Neurological Societies, testing for *LRRK2* mutations is indicated in patients with a history of dominant PD (Harbo et al., 2009). Sequencing of the coding region of the *LRRK2* gene revealed the p.G2019S mutation in our index patient (II.2). Both of his siblings (II.3 and II.4), as well as his son and daughter, also subsequently sought genetic testing for the familial p.G2019S mutation (Figure 6-1). Notably, family members should undergo direct testing of the known familial mutation in order to save costs. Although the patient's affected brother could be tested in the framework of establishing the (genetic) cause of his condition, the children (III.2 and III.3) have to undergo pre- and posttest counseling

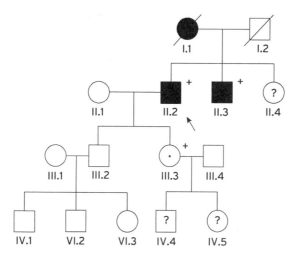

FIGURE 6-1 Pedigree of a patient with LRRK2-linked Parkinson disease. Males are represented by squares, females by circles. Diagonal lines through the symbols indicate deceased individuals. The index patient is marked with an arrow. The filled symbols mark affected family members. The plus symbols indicate the presence of the p.G2019S mutation in *LRRK2*. The dot symbolizes a nonmanifesting mutation carrier, the question marks indicate unknown mutational status.

by a human geneticist or authorized specialist/genetic counselor, as they were asymptomatic individuals. After genetic counseling, his unaffected sister (II.4) chose not to be tested. As the children in the fourth generation (IV.1-5) are asymptomatic minors, genetic testing was not considered appropriate.

If the genetic test for *LRRK2* mutations had been negative, alternative genes to consider for dominantly inherited PD would have been *VPS35* (Kumar et al., 2012) or *alpha-synuclein* (Table 6-1). The most common type of *alpha-synuclein* mutations are duplications, and duplication carriers may present with features entirely compatible with iPD (Kasten & Klein, 2013). As gene panels for PD and other neurodegenerative diseases are becoming increasingly available (and less expensive), a panel approach may be more economical and informative.

HOW DO YOU COUNSEL THE FAMILY?

LRRK2 mutations are dominantly inherited and thus the risk to any off-spring of an (affected or unaffected) mutation carrier to inherit the mutated

TABLE 6-1 **Autosomal dominant forms of Parkinson disease**

Designation	Phenotypic notes	Inheritance	Locus symbol
PARK-SNCA	Gene duplications: Classical PD. Missense mutations or gene triplications: Early-onset parkinsonism with prominent dementia.	AD	PARK1
PARK-LRRK2	Classical PD	AD	PARK8
PARK-VPS35	Classical PD	AD	PARK17

AD = autosomal dominant; PD = Parkinson disease.

allele is 50%. Due to the wide interindividual and intrafamilial variability of both penetrance and disease expression, no prediction can be made about who will become affected and to what extent. Genetic testing of the brother (II.3) confirmed the p.G2019S mutation as the likely cause of his PD. The patient's son (III.2) does not carry the mutation; thus, his children will also most likely be free of the mutation, as they only carry the general (extremely low) population risk of having inherited a *LRRK2* mutation from their mother or of harboring a de-novo mutation. The index patient's daughter (III.3), however, has inherited the familial pathogenic *LRRK2* mutation and the risk of having passed this on to her children is 50% for each child (IV.4 and IV.5). When the children reach the age of 18 years, they can choose to undergo presymptomatic testing after genetic counseling, if they so wish. The likelihood that the daughter (III.3), currently 35-years old will develop PD is 28% at age 59 years, 51% at 69 years, and 74% at 79 years (Healy et al., 2008).

HOW DO YOU TREAT DOMINANT PD?

Treatment of LRRK2-linked, as well as of other forms of dominantly inherited PD, is identical to that of iPD. It may include the entire spectrum of available therapeutic options including deep brain stimulation.

Further Reading

Harbo, H. F., Finsterer, J., Baets, J., Van Broeckhoven, C., Di Donato, S., Fontaine, B.,... & Gasset, T. (2009). EFNS guidelines on the molecular diagnosis of neurogenetic disorders: general issues, Huntington's disease, Parkinson's disease and dystonias. *European Journal of Neurology*, *16*(7), 777–785.

Healy, D. G., Falchi, M., O'Sullivan, S. S., Bonifati, V., Durr, A., Bressman, S.,... & Wood, N. W. (2008). Phenotype, genotype, and worldwide genetic penetrance of LRRK2-associated Parkinson's disease: A case-control study. *Lancet Neurology*, *7*(7), 583–590.

Kasten, M., & Klein, C. (2013). The many faces of alpha-synuclein mutations. *Movement Disorders*, *28*(6), 697–701.

Kumar, K. R., Lohmann, K., & Klein, C. (2012). Genetics of Parkinson disease and other movement disorders. *Current Opinions in Neurology*, *25*(4), 466–474.

Singleton, A. B., Farrer, M. J., & Bonifati, V. (2013). The genetics of Parkinson's disease: progress and therapeutic implications. *Movement Disorders*, *28*(1), 14–23.

7   Recessive Parkinson Disease

You are asked to see a 37-year-old self-employed furniture
designer with a four-year history of slowness of hand
movements, intermittent tremor of both hands, and muscle
stiffness, particularly of the right shoulder. Upon careful
history taking, the patient also reported cramping of the right
foot causing pain and difficulty walking long distances, which
preceded the other motor symptoms by about three years. The
motor problems have been slowly progressive and increasingly
interfering with the patient's work and family life as a father
of three small children. The patient had initially attributed
his problems to being overworked and only started seeking
medical attention in the past year. Despite having seen various
specialists, no definitive diagnosis was established and a
variety of possible conditions were discussed, ranging from
an orthopedic problem to "functional disease." The patient
additionally complained of a somewhat depressed mood and
anxiety related to his declining motor function. There was,
however, no deterioration of cognitive function and autonomic
function also remained normal. There was no family history of
parkinsonism or any other movement disorder; the patient's
parents were unrelated and he had one healthy sister aged
33 years.

Upon examination, there was mild hypomimia and
hypophonia, bradykinesia of fine finger and hand movements
bilaterally, more pronounced on the right, intermittent resting
tremor, and mild postural tremor of both hands, as well as
mild rigidity of the neck and at both elbow and wrist joints.
There was no postural instability. Stride length was reduced,
and the patient developed dystonic supination of the right foot
when walking up and down the corridor. Reflexes were brisk
but there were no pyramidal signs. The patient scored 24/108
points on the motor part of the Unified Parkinson's Disease
Rating Scale (UPDRS III) and 30/30 points on the Montreal
Cognitive Assessment (MoCA). The remainder of the neurological
examination was unremarkable.

What do you do now?

HOW DO YOU ESTABLISH A DIAGNOSIS OF RECESSIVE PARKINSON DISEASE?

As for any form of Parkinson disease (PD), the first diagnostic approach to genetic PD is clinical (Berardelli et al., 2013; Gelb et al., 1999). Although a definite diagnosis of PD can only be confirmed neuropathologically, and the neuropathological features of inherited PD are often different from those of the idiopathic form (iPD), the classic clinical triad of PD (brady-kinesia, resting tremor, and rigidity) with a good response to dopaminergic treatment is present in most patients with recessively inherited disease. Similar to iPD, tremor-dominant versus akinetic-rigid types also occur in monogenic disease (Pramstaller et al., 2005). Although there is no single clinical criterion distinguishing recessively inherited PD from iPD, there are a number of clinical features pointing to the presence of possible *Parkin* mutations, which are by far the most common known cause of recessive PD. These "red flags" include a significantly earlier and more symmetrical onset, dystonia (sometimes also as presenting sign) and hyperreflexia, slower progression of the disease, and a tendency toward a greater response to levodopa despite lower doses (Hedrich et al., 2004). Another important feature of Parkin-linked disease is that cognitive decline or dementia occurs only rarely, and is not more common in *Parkin* mutation carriers than in the general population (Grünewald et al., 2013).

Family history is often negative in patients with recessive PD, especially when they originate from a population with a low degree of consanguinity and when families are small in size. The frequency of (heterozygous) *Parkin* mutations in the general population is estimated at about 1–3%. Statistically, 1 in 4 offspring of two heterozygous mutation carriers will be a compound-heterozygous mutation carrier (harboring different *Parkin* mutations on each of the two alleles) and become affected (Figure 7-1). In populations with a high degree of consanguinity, patients usually carry homozygous mutations (the same *Parkin* mutation on both alleles).

Given the typical features of recessive PD (early onset below the age of 35 years, slow progression, presence of dystonia and hyperreflexia, and absence of cognitive decline), genetic testing for genes causing recessive PD is indicated even in patients with a negative family history (Harbo et al.,

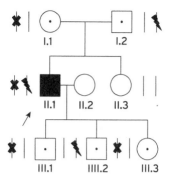

FIGURE 7-1 Pedigree of a patient with Parkin-linked Parkinson disease. Males are represented by squares, females by circles. The index patient is marked with an arrow. The filled symbol marks the only affected family member. The dots symbolizes nonmanifesting heterozygous mutation carriers. Each of the parents (I.1 and I.2) and all three children carry one mutated *Parkin* allele (a deletion of exon three [del ex 3] or a point mutation [c.924C>T]). Alleles are represented by vertical lines; mutations by a cross and a lightning bolt, respectively. The affected family member has inherited both (different) mutations in the *Parkin* gene and is therefore compound-heterozygous for *Parkin* mutations. His sister (II.2) has inherited the normal allele from both of their parents and is unaffected by Parkinson disease.

2009). Genetic testing in the index patient confirmed the presence of compound-heterozygous *Parkin* mutations (Figure 7-1). Based on mutation frequency, *Parkin* mutations are the first gene to consider, followed by mutations in *PINK1* or *DJ-1*. Genetic testing for mutations in these genes is increasingly offered as a panel, which may reduce costs and turn-around time of the test.

There are a number of other recessively inherited, atypical forms of parkinsonism (as opposed to "recessive Parkinson disease," which clinically closely resembles iPD). These conditions usually manifest in adolescence and are accompanied by a variety of unusual neurological features (e.g., early cognitive decline, supranuclear gaze palsy, pyramidal or cerebellar features) that are not found in recessive PD caused by mutations in *Parkin, PINK1* or *DJ-1* (Table 7-1).

Importantly, genetic testing for all three of these genes should comprise not only sequence analysis but also quantitative testing, which is usually performed by multiplex ligation-dependent analysis (MLPA). MLPA is able

TABLE 7-1 **Autosomal recessive forms of Parkinson disease**

Designation	Phenotypic notes	Locus symbol
Early-onset Parkinson disease		
PARK-PARKIN	Relatively benign course, good and sustained response to dopaminergic treatment, dystonia frequently at onset, no dementia	PARK2
PARK-PINK1		PARK6
PARK-DJ1		PARK7
Atypical, juvenile parkinsonism or complex phenotypes		
PARK-ATP13A2	**Kufor-Rakeb syndrome (supranuclear gaze palsy, dementia, pyramidal signs, poor long-term response to dopaminergic treatment)**	PARK9
PARK-FBX07	Early onset parkinsonism with pyramidal signs	PARK15
PARK-DNAJC6	Mental retardation and seizures may be part of the phenotypic spectrum	PARK19
PARK-SYNJ1	Seizures, cognitive decline, abnormal eye movements, and dystonia may be part of the phenotypic spectrum	PARK20

to detect deletions and duplications of entire exons, an important type of mutation in recessive PD. For example, in Parkin-linked disease, such gene dosage changes account for at least 50% of all mutations and would be overlooked by isolated sequence analysis.

HOW DO YOU COUNSEL THE FAMILY?

Parkin (as well as *PINK1* and *DJ-1*) mutations are recessively inherited with full penetrance. Mean age of onset in most populations is in the mid-30s, however, cases with juvenile onset or with late onset in the 60s or even 70s have also been described. Despite interindividual (and intra-familial) variability, counseling of affected individuals should include a discussion of the relatively benign course of the disease with a good and sustained treatment response, as well as the very low likelihood of developing dementia (Brüggemann & Klein, [Internet]. 2013; Grünewald et al., 2013).

The risk to the patient's sister (II.3) to inherit both *Parkin* mutations from her parents and thus to develop Parkin-linked PD is 25%. If she requests genetic testing, as in our case, she needs to undergo pre- and posttest genetic counseling by a human geneticist or authorized specialist, as she is asymptomatic. The parents each carry one of the mutations in the heterozygous state, resulting in a risk to their offspring to also be a heterozygous carrier of 50%. An average of 25% of the children will have no mutations (as in II.3, the patient's sister), and two mutations are transmitted to the remaining 25% (as in II.1, our index case). All three of our index patient's children inherited one of the two mutated alleles. Given that their mutational status can be predicted based on the pedigree structure and, importantly, they are asymptomatic minors, genetic testing is not indicated. Their risk to develop PD is extremely low and would only have to be considered for counseling in the unlikely event that their mother (individual II.2) also happened to be a *Parkin* mutation carrier, which is not the case in our family. Importantly, however, this latter scenario needs to be considered in consanguineous families and should be included in the family's counseling.

HOW DO YOU TREAT RECESSIVE PD?

Treatment of Parkin-linked as well as PINK1- and DJ-1-linked PD is not different from that of iPD. Due to the early onset and expected very long duration of treatment, often for several decades, it may be advisable to delay levodopa treatment because of the risk of dyskinesias. However, patients need to be advised about the risk of impulse control disorders as a side effect of dopamine agonists. Finally, patients with recessive PD have been shown to respond well to deep brain stimulation.

Further Reading

Berardelli, A., Wenning, G. K., Antonini, A., Berg, D., Bloem, B. R., Bonifati, V.,...& Vidailhet, M. (2013). EFNS/MDS-ES/ENS [corrected] recommendations for the diagnosis of Parkinson's disease. *European Journal of Neurology, 20*(1), 16–34.

Brüggemann, N., & Klein, C. (2013). Parkin type of early-onset Parkinson disease. In R. A. Pagon, M. P. Adam, T. D. Bird, et al., (Eds.) *GeneReviews™ [Internet].* Seattle, WA: University of Washington, 1993-2014. (http://www.ncbi.nlm.nih.gov/books/NBK1478/)

Gelb, D. J., Oliver, E., & Gilman, S. (1999). Diagnostic criteria for Parkinson disease. *Archives in Neurology, 56*(1), 33–39.

Grünewald, A., Kasten, M., Ziegler, A., & Klein, C. (2013). Next-generation phenotyping using the parkin example: time to catch up with genetics. *JAMA Neurology, 70*(9), 1186–1191.

Harbo, H. F., Finsterer, J., Baets, J., Van Broeckhoven, C., Di Donato, S., Fontaine, B.,...& Gasser, T. (2009). EFNS guidelines on the molecular diagnosis of neurogenetic disorders: general issues, Huntington's disease, Parkinson's disease and dystonias. *European Journal of Neurology, 16*(7), 777–785.

Hedrich, K., Eskelson, C., Wilmot, B., Marder, K., Harris, J., Garrels, J.,...& Kramer, P. (2004). Distribution, type, and origin of Parkin mutations: review and case studies. *Movement Disorders, 19*(10), 1146–1157.

Pramstaller, P. P., Schlossmacher, M. G., Jacques, T. S., Scaravilli, F., Eskelson, C., Pepivani, I.,...& Klein, C. (2005). Lewy body Parkinson's disease in a large pedigree with 77 Parkin mutation carriers. *Annals of Neurology, 58*(3), 411–422.

8 Gaucher Disease and Parkinson Disease

You see a 41-year-old man from Serbia with early onset Parkinson disease (EOPD) in your movement disorder clinic. His symptoms started at the age of 39 years and the signs at presentation included left-sided rigidity and bradykinesia. He has not responded well to levodopa therapy. His family history is negative for neurological disorders.

On examination, he has signs of parkinsonism such as rigidity, bradykinesia, and a rest tremor. His signs are asymmetrical with the left side being more affected.

You calculate the motor part of the Unified Parkinson's Disease Rating Scale III as 40/108. He has a score of 1.5 (both on and off treatment) for the Hoehn and Yahr Scale. You also assess his cognition as 26/30 on the Mini-Mental State Examination.

He is enrolled in a study (Kumar et al., 2013) in which we performed Sanger sequencing to screen Serbian PD patients for common mutations in the *glucocerebrosidase* (*GBA*) gene. He was found to have the N370S mutation as well as the D409H;H255Q double mutant allele.

What do you do now?

It appears that the patient is a compound heterozygote for mutations in the *GBA* gene. However, we cannot confirm that both alleles of *GBA* gene are affected through Sanger sequencing alone, and his parents were not available for genetic testing. If the patient is a compound heterozygote, he is at risk of developing other clinical manifestations of Gaucher disease.

Gaucher disease can lead to a spectrum of clinical findings ranging from being asymptomatic to a perinatal lethal disorder. There are 3 major clinical types (types 1, 2, and 3) and two other subtypes (perinatal-lethal and cardiovascular, Pastores & Hughes, 1993).

Type 1 Gaucher disease is referred to as the non-neuronopathic form of Gaucher disease because the central nervous system is said to be spared. The features of this condition range from mild to severe, and onset may be from childhood to adulthood. The clinical features include hepatosplenomegaly, anemia, thrombocytopenia, lung disease, and bony abnormalities such as osteopenia, focal lytic or sclerotic lesions, and osteonecrosis.

Types 2 and 3 of Gaucher disease are known as neuronopathic forms of the disorder because, in comparison to type 1, they tend to affect the central nervous system. In additional to the clinical features of type 1, they also cause additional neurological manifestations including abnormal eye movements, seizures, spasticity, myoclonus, and dementia. Disease with onset prior to two years of age, with limited psychomotor development, and a rapidly progressive course with death by age two to four years can be classified as Gaucher disease type 2. Individuals with Gaucher disease type 3 may also have onset before 2 years of age, but usually have a more slowly progressive course, with survival into the third or fourth decade. The perinatal-lethal form is characterized by ichthyosiform or collodion skin abnormalities or with nonimmune hydrops fetalis. The cardiovascular form is characterized by calcification of the aortic and mitral valves, mild splenomegaly, corneal opacities, and supranuclear ophthalmoplegia.

Mutations in *GBA* can be categorized into three groups, based on their deduced and observed phenotypic effects (Beutler et al., 2005). For example, the N370S mutation can be classified as a 'mild' mutation, and individuals with at least one N370S allele are unlikely to develop neuronopathic forms. It is also important to note that the H255Q mutation often occurs in *cis* with the D409H mutation, as seen in the patient from the clinical vignette.

It has now become apparent that Gaucher disease and PD are linked, starting with observations that patients with Gaucher disease (and their relatives) appeared to be at risk of parkinsonism. Larger studies confirmed that *GBA* mutations (even a single mutation, including the N370S mutation) are associated with PD. (Sidransky et al., 2009). In fact, about 5–10% of patients with PD will have at least one *GBA* mutation. This effect is apparent across different ethnic groups (including the Serbian population, as shown in our study). Patients with *GBA*-associated PD have a similar clinical phenotype to PD patients without *GBA* mutations, although mutation carriers tend to present earlier, are more likely to have a family history of PD, and tend to have more cognitive changes. Mutations in the *GBA* gene have previously been considered a risk factor for PD; however, the penetrance is relatively high, and so perhaps, *GBA* should be considered a dominant causal gene (Anheim et al., 2012). It is likely that the *GBA* mutations identified in the patient from the clinical vignette contributed to the development of EOPD.

The patient was re-evaluated to assess for manifestations of Gaucher disease, and was found to have anemia, thrombocytopenia, and splenomegaly. He was referred to a specialty Gaucher disease unit for management of complications of Gaucher disease and consideration of enzyme replacement therapy.

KEY POINTS TO REMEMBER ABOUT GAUCHER DISEASE AND PARKINSON DISEASE

- Gaucher disease is caused by mutations in the *glucocerebrosidase* (*GBA*) and there are a range of clinical findings, with three major clinical types (type 1, 2, and 3) and two other subtypes (perinatal-lethal and cardiovascular).
- Mutations in the *GBA* gene are also associated with Parkinson disease (PD).
- Patients with *GBA*-associated PD have a similar clinical phenotype to PD patients without *GBA* mutations, although mutation carriers tend to present earlier, are more likely to have a family history of PD, and tend to have more cognitive changes.

Further Reading

Anheim, M., Elbaz, A., Lesage, S., Durr, A., Condroyer, C., Viallet, F.,... & Brice, A. (2012). Penetrance of Parkinson disease in glucocerebrosidase gene mutation carriers. *Neurology, 78,* 417–420.

Beutler, E., Gelbart, T., & Scott, C. R. (2005). Hematologically important mutations: Gaucher disease. *Blood Cells, Molecules & Diseases, 35,* 355–364.

Kumar, K. R., Ramirez, A., Göbel, A., Kresojevic, N., Svetel, M., Lohmann, K.,... & Grünewald, A. (2013). Glucocerebrosidase mutations in a Serbian Parkinson's disease population. *European Journal of Neurology, 20,* 402–405.

Pastores, G. M. & Hughes, D. A. (1993). Gaucher disease. In R. A. Pagon, M. P. Adam, T. D. Bird, C. R. Dolan, C. T. Fong, & K. Stephens (Eds.) *GeneReviews.* Seattle WA.

Sidransky, E., Nalls, M. A., Aasly, J. O., Aharon-Peretz, J., Annesi, G., Barbosa, E. R.,... & Ziegler, S. G. (2009). Multicenter analysis of glucocerebrosidase mutations in Parkinson's disease. *New England Journal of Medicine, 361,* 1651–1661.

9   Spinocerebellar Ataxia Type 2

A 54-year-old man presents to your clinic with a progressive cerebellar ataxia syndrome in the company of his mother. His mother recalls that he had poor balance since the age of 50 years. He has had recurrent falls over the past year and has also noticed slurring of his speech. On specific questioning, his mother wonders if his memory is impaired. He has not noticed any weakness or sensory symptoms in his limbs and his bowel and bladder function is intact.

On examination, he has mild dysarthria. His saccadic eye movements were abnormally slowed indicating oculomotor impairment. He also has a tremor of the chin. The tone, power, and reflexes in the upper limbs are normal. However, there is obvious dysmetria on finger-nose testing and dysdiadochokinesis for both arms. For the lower limb examination, the tone and power were normal, but there was evidence of hyperreflexia and heel-shin ataxia. His gait was broad-based and ataxic. There were no signs of parkinsonism.

He had a normal birth. He did not walk until the age of 17 months and he only started to speak by the age of two years, which was a little slower than his siblings.

His past medical history included type 2 diabetes mellitus, hypertension, and depression treated with metformin, ramipril, and citalopram, respectively. His alcohol intake was not excessive.

From the family history, it is apparent that neither his parents nor his four siblings had any neurological symptoms, although his father died at a relatively young age from a motor vehicle accident.

What do you do now?

The patient presents with progressive cerebellar ataxia with possible signs of corticospinal tract involvement (e.g., lower limb hyperreflexia) and may be considered to have a spastic-ataxia type phenotype. The differential diagnosis in this circumstance is extensive.

In the first instance, acquired and potentially reversible causes should be excluded. Acquired causes include structural or vascular pontocerebellar abnormalities, inflammatory central nervous system diseases (e.g., multiple sclerosis), superficial siderosis, paraneoplastic syndromes, vitamin deficiencies (e.g., vitamin E, vitamin B12, copper), toxins, and adverse effects from medications (such as phenytoin; de Bot, Willemsen, Vermeer, Kremer, & van de Warrenburg, 2012).

There are many different genetic causes of spastic-ataxia phenotypes with different modes of inheritance. The classification of these disorders can be confusing for clinicians. Inherited causes of spastic-ataxia include the spinocerebellar ataxias (SCAs), autosomal recessive ataxia of Charlevoix-Saguenay (ARSACS), Friedreich ataxia (see chapter 12, this volume), cerebrotendinous xanthomatosis, and hereditary spastic paraplegias with signs of ataxia (e.g., SPG7; de Bot et al., 2012).

Many different SCA loci (SCA1-36) have been identified (Rub et al., 2012). The term *autosomal dominant cerebellar ataxia* (ADCA) can be applied to the CAG-repeat or polyglutamine ataxias, (e.g., SCA1, SCA2, SCA3, SCA6, SCA7, SCA17, and dentatorubral-pallidoluysian atrophy). Of these, SCA1, SCA2, SCA3, SCA6, and SCA7 constitute the most frequent causes of ADCA, accounting for 50–60% of all families affected by ADCA globally (Rub et al., 2013). These SCAs share a similar clinical phenotype, which is characterized by gradual and predominantly adult disease-onset, a progressive worsening of cerebellar and noncerebellar symptoms, and average disease duration of 15–30 years (Rub et al., 2013).

The patient had a cerebral magnetic resonance imaging (MRI) study to investigate for structural and vascular causes. The MRI showed evidence of marked atrophy in the cerebellar hemispheres and brainstem (Figure 9-1).

It was decided that the patient should be screened for the most common genetically defined ADCAs (Table 9-1).

Other laboratory investigations such as antineuronal antibodies and vitamin E levels were normal.

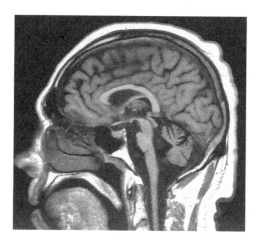

FIGURE 9-1 Brain MRI (sagittal) from the patient demonstrating evidence of ponto-cerebellar atrophy.

TABLE 9-1 **Results of testing for the most common genetically defined autosomal dominant cerebellar ataxias**

Condition	Gene	Result	Normal range
SCA1	*ATXN1*	Allele 1: 31 repeats Allele 2: 31 repeats (presumed homozygous)	Normal range: 24–38 repeats Affected range: 42–82 repeats
SCA2	*ATXN2*	Allele 1: 22 repeats Allele 2: 38 repeats	Normal range: 17–31 repeats Intermediate range: 31–34 repeats Affected range: 35–52 repeats
SCA3/ Machado- Joseph disease	*ATXN3*	Allele 1: 23 repeats Allele 2: 23 repeats (presumed homozygous)	Normal range: <44 repeats Affected range: 52–86 repeats
SCA6	*CACNA1A*	Allele 1: 13 repeats Allele 2: 13 repeats (presumed homozygous)	Normal range: ≤18 repeats Affected range: 20–33 repeats
SCA7	*ATXN7*	Allele 1: 10 repeats Allele 2: 12 repeats	Normal range: ≤19 repeats Affected range: ≥36 repeats

The abnormal result is highlighted in gray. SCA = spinocerebellar ataxia.

The results suggest the patient has SCA2. The typical clinical phenotype of SCA2 is a "cerebellar plus" syndrome, with progressive ataxia, dysarthria, dysphagia, oculomotor impairment (e.g., early and severe slowing of saccades), action and postural tremor, peripheral neuropathy (with early areflexia of the upper limbs), autonomic dysfunction, sleep disturbance, executive dysfunction, and cognitive decline (Rub et al., 2013). It can also present with a levodopa-responsive akinetic-rigid syndrome that resembles Parkinson disease. Spinocerebellar ataxia 2 is commonly seen in adulthood, but the age at onset correlates with the length of the expanded CAG-repeat in the mutated allele. Moreover, the clinical phenotype may be especially severe (e.g., with retinitis pigmentosa, myoclonus-epilepsy and early onset parkinsonism) in those with more than 200 CAG repeats and also in patients with homozygous mutations (Rub et al., 2013).

The phenotype for the patient in the clinical vignette would be consistent with an ADCA, although there are no features that strongly suggestive the diagnosis of SCA2 in particular (e.g., levodopa-responsive parkinsonism). The patient did not have a positive family history, but this may be explained by the fact that the patient's father died before developing symptoms, or it may be due to pronounced anticipation which is a feature of SCA2 (Rub et al., 2013).

It is important to note that some authors have suggested alternative diagnostic strategies for sporadic patients presenting with a spastic-ataxia phenotype, such as testing for SPG7, ARSACS, and Friedreich ataxia in the first instance.

Symptomatic treatments (such as a physiotherapy assessment) are the mainstay of management in this patient since there are no treatments that target the underlying disease process.

KEY POINTS TO REMEMBER ABOUT SPINOCEREBELLAR ATAXIA TYPE 2

- It is important to exclude acquired causes first (e.g., structural or vascular pontocerebellar abnormalities) prior to considering an inherited ataxia.
- The causes of a spastic-ataxia phenotype are varied and include spinocerebellar ataxias (SCAs), autosomal recessive ataxia of Charlevoix-Saguenay (ARSACS), Friedreich ataxia, cerebrotendinous

xanthomatosis, and hereditary spastic paraplegias with signs of ataxia (e.g., SPG7).

- Common autosomal dominant cerebellar ataxias (ADCAs) include SCA1, SCA2, SCA3, SCA6 and SCA7 and are characterized by gradual and predominantly adult disease onset, and a progressive worsening of cerebellar and noncerebellar symptoms.
- The typical clinical phenotype of SCA2 is a "cerebellar plus" syndrome, with progressive ataxia, dysarthria, dysphagia, oculomotor impairment (e.g., early and severe slowing of saccades), action and postural tremor, peripheral neuropathy (with early areflexia of the upper limbs), autonomic dysfunction, sleep disturbance, executive dysfunction, cognitive decline, and levodopa-responsive parkinsonism.

Further Reading

de Bot, S. T., Willemsen, M. A., Vermeer, S., Kremer, H. P., & van de Warrenburg, B. P. (2012). Reviewing the genetic causes of spastic-ataxias. *Neurology, 79*, 1507–1514.

Rub, U., Schols, L., Paulson, H., Auburger, G., Kermer, P., Jen, J. C.,...& Deller, T. (2013). Clinical features, neurogenetics and neuropathology of the polyglutamine spinocerebellar ataxias type 1, 2, 3, 6 and 7. *Progress in Neurobiology, 104*, 38–66.

10 Spinocerebellar Ataxia Type 17

A 42-year-old man of Asian descent is referred to your neurogenetics clinic. He has a 6-year history of difficulty with gait and balance that has been getting progressively worse over the last two years. He also reports a mild action tremor of the arms, which has been present for the past 15–20 years. Approximately nine years ago he was investigated with magnetic resonance imaging (MRI) of the brain for light-headedness on standing, which revealed an incidental finding of marked cerebellar atrophy involving both cerebellar hemispheres and the vermis. Three years ago he was admitted to a local hospital with episodes of confusion associated with automatisms. He was initially treated with sodium valproate, which failed to control his seizures and was later changed to lamotrigine. More recently, his sister has noticed that his speech has become slurred. He has also had problems with short-term memory loss and experienced difficulty with multitasking. There is no family history of ataxia or other neurological disease.

On examination, his blood pressure was 105/70 with no postural drop. His speech is dysarthric. There was mild gaze-evoked nystagmus bilaterally and saccadic intrusions into smooth pursuit eye movements. There was mild spasticity in the upper and lower limbs. Power in the arms and legs was normal, and reflexes were generally brisk. Hoffman and Babinski signs were negative. He has a mild intention tremor in the upper limbs and mild heel-shin ataxia in the lower limbs. He walks with a wide-based, unsteady gait. There was no chorea or other hyperkinetic movements.

What do you do now?

This gentleman presents with several features including a progressive ataxia syndrome with mild corticospinal tract signs, seizures, and cognitive impairment. You begin to wonder whether the patient could have a type of spinocerebellar ataxia (SCA) given that he has a phenotype of slowly progressive ataxia in conjunction with evidence of cerebellar atrophy on neuroimaging. In this case, his mode of inheritance is unclear, the onset of symptoms is in adulthood, and the patient may still have an autosomal dominant condition given the reduced penetrance that occurs in many of the SCAs.

You first order laboratory investigations, including autoantibodies to celiac disease and vitamin E levels, which are normal.

You consider whether the patient could have an autosomal dominant cerebellar ataxia (ADCA), such as SCA1, 2, 3, 6, 7, 17 and dentatorubral-pallidoluysian atrophy or DRLPA, which can lead to an adult onset of slowly progressive cerebellar and noncerebellar features, and so you order some genetic tests (Table 10-1).

Testing for SCA17 shows one allele with 47 CAG/CAA repeats, which is outside the normal range. An individual with an allele in this range may or may not develop symptoms of SCA17 (i.e., reduced penetrance). It is important to note that many conditions can present with sporadic, progressive ataxic phenotypes, and alternative diagnostic strategies have been suggested (deBot, Willemsen, Vermeer, Kremer, & van de Warrenburg, 2012).

Features of SCA17 include ataxia, dementia, seizures, and involuntary movements such as chorea and dystonia (DeMichele et al., 2003). Psychiatric symptoms, corticospinal tract signs, and rigidity are also common (Toyshima, Onodera, Yamada, Tsuji, & Takahashi, 1993). The age of onset varies from 3–55 years. The disorder often presents with ataxia and psychiatric manifestations followed by involuntary movement, parkinsonism, dementia, and corticospinal signs. Typical findings on MRI of the brain include atrophy of the cerebrum, brain stem, and cerebellum. It is important to note that the clinical features typically correlate with the length of the repeat expansion, although they are not absolutely predictive of the clinical course. It is also notable that SCA17 can cause a Huntington disease

TABLE 10-1 **Results of genetic testing for some of the autosomal dominant cerebellar ataxias**

Condition	Gene	Result	Normal range
SCA1	*ATXN1*	Allele 1: 28 repeats Allele 2: 30 repeats	Normal range: 24–38 repeats Affected range: 42–82 repeats
SCA2	*ATXN2*	Allele 1: 22 repeats Allele 2: 22 repeats (presumed homozygous)	Normal range: 17–31 repeats Intermediate range: 31–34 repeats Affected range: 35–52 repeats
SCA3/ Machado- Joseph disease	*ATXN3*	Allele 1: 14 repeats Allele 2: 30 repeats	Normal range: <44 repeats Affected range: 52–86 repeats
SCA6	*CACNA1A*	Allele 1: 11 repeats Allele 2: 13 repeats	Normal range: ≤18 repeats Affected range: 20–33 repeats
SCA7	*ATXN7*	Allele 1: 10 repeats Allele 2: 10 repeats (presumed homozygous)	Normal range: ≤19 repeats Affected range: ≥36 repeats
SCA17	*TBP*	Allele 1: 47 Allele 2: 36	Affected range: ≥49 repeats. Reduced penetrance: 41–48 repeats Normal range: 25–40 repeats.

The abnormal result is highlighted in gray. SCA = spinocerebellar ataxia.

phenocopy syndrome (Huntington disease-like 4 or HDL4, see chapter 5, this volume) as well as Parkinson disease-like, Creutzfeldt-Jakob disease-like and Alzheimer disease-like phenotypes (Stevanin & Brice, 2008).

You provide the patient with genetic counseling and continue to see the patient for management of his seizures. You also refer the patient for a neuropsychological evaluation which reveals compromised neurocognitive function for language, visuospatial perception, mental processing speed, psychomotor control and memory capacity.

Further Reading

de Bot, S. T., Willemsen, M. A., Vermeer, S., Kremer, H. P., & van de Warrenburg, B. P. (2012). Reviewing the genetic causes of spastic-ataxias. *Neurology*, 79, 1507–1514.

De Michele, G., Maltecca, F., Carella, M., Volpe, G., Orio, M., De Falco, A.,...& Bruni, A. (2003). Dementia, ataxia, extrapyramidal features, and epilepsy: phenotype spectrum in two Italian families with spinocerebellar ataxia type 17. *Neurological Sciences*, 24, 166–167.

Stevanin, G., & Brice, A. (2008). Spinocerebellar ataxia 17 (SCA17) and Huntington's disease-like 4 (HDL4). *Cerebellum*, 7, 170–178.

Toyoshima, Y., Onodera, O., Yamada, M., Tsuji, S., & Takahashi, H. (1993). Spinocerebellar ataxia type 17. In R. A. Pagon, M. P. Adam, T. D. Bird, C. R. Dolan, C. T. Fong, & K. Stephens (Eds.), *GeneReviews*. Seattle, WA: University of Washington.

11 Sialidosis

You are referred a 28-year-old man with a history of an ataxic disorder.

His symptoms started 10 years ago, when he started falling over while playing ball sports. Since then, his balance has become progressively worse. In particular, he notices difficulty on uneven ground or when he is tired. He also observes that his speech becomes slurred when attempting multisyllabic words during oral presentations at work. He has noticed difficulty with fine finger movements, although he has retained the ability to play a guitar. He has trouble focusing with his eyes when he is tired, but has no other visual symptoms.

On examination, the visual acuity is 6/9 with glasses, and visual fields are normal with no visual inattention. The extraocular eye movements were also normal. Dilated fundoscopy performed together with a neuro-ophthalmologist reveals the following finding (Figure 11-1).

He has mild dysmetria on finger-nose testing, heel-shin ataxia and unsteadiness on tandem gait. There is normal tone, power, and reflexes in the upper limbs. The lower limbs also show normal tone and power with downgoing plantars, although hyperreflexia is evident. Sensory modalities are intact.

In terms of the family history, the patient is one of five siblings (Figure 11-2). His eldest brother (II.1) also has an ataxic disorder with progressive gait difficulties since the age of 16 years, which led to him being restricted to a wheelchair for mobility by his fourth decade. Additional neurological manifestations in the brother include myoclonus and generalized seizures. His younger sister (II.5) is also affected by a similar disorder.

What do you do now?

You note that the patient has a small, circular choroid shape in the fovea centralis, suggestive of a cherry red spot. A cherry red spot has several causes including central retinal artery occlusion and metabolic storage diseases such as Tay-Sachs disease, Sandhoff disease, Niemann-Pick disease, Fabry disease, Gaucher disease, and sialidosis (mucolipidosis type I; Heroman, Rychwalski, & Barr, 2008).

The presence of an ataxic disorder in both affected siblings and myoclonic epilepsy in the patient's brother is suggestive of the cherry red spot-myoclonus syndrome (sialidosis type 1). Sialdosis is a rare autosomal recessive disorder resulting from mutations in the *NEU1* gene (Lai et al., 2009; O'Brien, 1978). It is characterized by deficiency of α-*N*-acetylneuraminidase (sialidase) in leukocytes and cultured fibroblasts, leading to intracellular accumulation of excess sialyloligosaccharides. This is histologically observed as abnormal vacuolization of various cell types. Patients with type I disease usually develop symptoms of myoclonic epilepsy, visual problems, and ataxia in the second or the third decade of life, with macular cherry red spots always present. A severe infantile form of sialidosis (type II) also exists and is characterized by coarse facies, hepatolomegaly, bony changes of dysostosis multiplex, and developmental delay.

In this patient, you order magnetic resonance imaging (MRI) of the brain and spinal cord, which did not reveal any structural lesions. Urine oligosaccharide analysis with thin layer chromatography was clearly abnormal in the patient and consistent with neuramindase deficiency due to sialidosis. Furthermore, neuraminidase activity was not detectable in the patients

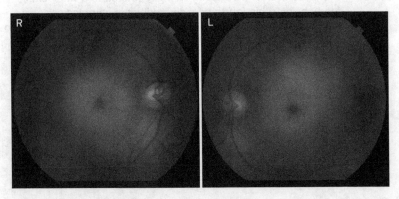

FIGURE 11-1 Fundoscopic pictures of the right (R) and left (L) eye showing bilateral cherry red spots.

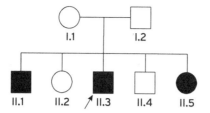

FIGURE 11-2 Pedigree of a family with ataxia, myoclonic epilepsy, and retinal changes. Males are represented by squares, females by circles. The index patient is indicated with an arrow. Filled symbols mark affected individuals.

cultured skin fibroblasts. The patients β-galactosidase was normal, which excluded the diagnosis of galactosialidosis, which also presents with reduced neuraminidase activity. Genetic testing for spinocerebellar ataxia type 1, 2, 3, 6, and 7 was negative, as was testing for Friedreich ataxia type 1.

You inform the patient about the diagnosis of sialidosis type 1 and provide genetic counseling. You continue to see the patient in clinic for symptomatic management; however, there are no disease modifying therapies available.

KEY POINTS TO REMEMBER ABOUT SIALIDOSIS

- Fundoscopic examination can give important clues to the diagnosis in patients with inherited neurological conditions.
- A cherry red spot can be caused by central retinal artery occlusion and metabolic storage diseases such as Tay-Sachs disease, Sandhoff disease, Niemann-Pick disease, Fabry disease, Gaucher disease, and sialidosis.
- Sialodisis is an autosomal recessive disorder resulting from mutations in the *NEU1* gene and is characterized by the deficiency of α-*N*-acetylneuraminidase (sialidase) in leukocytes and cultured fibroblasts.
- Type 1 sialodisis (cherry red spot-myoclonus syndrome) manifests with symptoms of myoclonic epilepsy, visual problems, and ataxia in the second or the third decade of life and macular cherry red spots are always present.
- A severe infantile form of sialidosis (type II) also exists and is characterized by coarse facies, hepatolomegaly, bony changes of dysostosis multiplex, and developmental delay.

Further Reading

Heroman, J. W., Rychwalski, P., & Barr, C. C. (2008). Cherry red spot in sialidosis (mucolipidosis type I). *Archives of ophthalmology, 126,* 270–271.

Lai, S. C., Chen, R. S., Wu Chou, Y. H., Chang, H. C., Kao L. Y., Huang, Y. Z., ... & Lu, C. S. A longitudinal study of Taiwanese sialidosis type 1: An insight into the concept of cherry-red spot myoclonus syndrome. European Journal of Neurology, *16,* 912–919.

O'Brien, J. S. (1978). The cherry red spot-myoclonus syndrome: A newly recognized inherited lysosomal storage disease due to acid neuraminidase deficiency. *Clinical Genetics, 14,* 55–60.

12 Friedreich Ataxia

A 10-year-old boy accompanied by his father presents to the emergency department because of hyperglycemia noted by the local pediatrician. During history taking, it is becoming clear that the boy has a long-standing history of unexplained neurological problems since early childhood. After an uneventful birth and normal early development, he experienced difficulty walking from the age of 3 years. He became slightly unsteady on his feet and developed a tendency to walk on his toes. In spite of intense physiotherapy his symptoms deteriorated. Around the age of 8 years his fine finger movements became clumsy. Also, he developed progressive lateral curvature of the spine. The patient has a 7-year-old sister who is healthy and his family history is unremarkable.

On examination, there are no neuropsychiatric abnormalities. He has mild right-sided scoliosis with the trunk tilted to the left and the left shoulder slightly drooped and rotated forward. There are no other skeletal changes or skin lesions. Ocular pursuit is saccadic but the range of horizontal and vertical eye movements is normal. The vestibular-ocular reflex (VOR) is normal bilaterally but fixation suppression of the VOR is incomplete. There is generalized and symmetric hypotonia, equinovarus deformity of both feet and symmetric mild distal weakness. The tendon reflexes are absent but plantar responses are extensor bilaterally. Joint position sense and vibration sensation are impaired and there are mild pseudo-athetoid movements when holding out the arms. There is dysmetria on finger-to-nose testing and there is also evidence of dysdiadochokinesia. Heel-to-shin testing reveals leg ataxia. His walking is wide-based ataxic with impaired postural stability. He has dysarthria with scanning speech.

What do you do now?

The clinical syndrome suggests involvement of the pyramidal tract, fast conducting sensory neurons and cerebellar pathways. In addition, there is scoliosis and signs of systemic disease. Given that gait problems were the earliest and remain the most prominent clinical feature, the boy's disease can be placed in the spectrum of early onset progressive ataxias. This is a large group of neurodegenerative disorders comprising predominantly autosomal recessive diseases. Autosomal recessive cerebellar ataxia should be considered in patients younger than 30 years of age with a persistent and gradually worsening gait or balance disorder.

Although many different causes have to be considered, Friedreich ataxia (FA) is by far the most common. In fact, it is the most common hereditary ataxia overall with a prevalence of approximately 1/30,000 to 1/50,000 in most populations and a carrier frequency of approximately 1/85 in the Caucasian population.

Onset age typically ranges between 5 and 25 years. Progressive trunk and limb ataxia, dysarthria, and muscle weakness are almost invariably present. Ataxia, the clinical hallmark in FA, is due to a combination of cerebellar and spinocerebellar degeneration and sensory neuronopathy. The latter leads to areflexia and impaired vibration sense and proprioception. It is also the basis of degeneration of the posterior columns of the spinal cord. Oculomotor abnormalities include square wave jerks, saccadic pursuit, fixation problems, pathological VOR, impaired VOR suppression or both. Scoliosis, pes cavus, and equinovarus deformity are present in many patients (Figure 12-1).

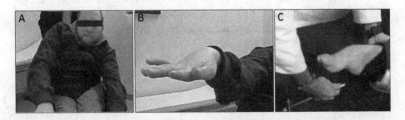

FIGURE 12-1 Typical signs of advanced Friedreich ataxia in two wheelchair-bound patients. A. A patient is shown strapped to the wheelchair to prevent truncal instability caused by severe right-sided scoliosis accompanied by shortening of the trunk, left shoulder droop and left hip elevation. B. When holding out the arms, there is finger and wrist posturing due to severely impaired joint position sense. C. A pes cavus deformity is shown.

Patients with FA often show abnormal speech understanding when tested with levels of background noise typical of everyday listening conditions. Recent studies of neuropsychological function also suggest reduced verbal fluency and information processing speed, visuo-spatial deficits, and difficulties with attention and working memory in FA.

On neuroimaging, cerebellar and cervical spinal cord atrophy may be observed.

Importantly, cardiomyopathy is present in most FA patients. This can be asymptomatic but may lead to signs of heart failure, palpitations, and sudden death due to cardiac arrhythmias. Investigations of cardiac function are usually abnormal with several common findings including T-wave inversion, left-axis deviation, and repolarization abnormalities on electrocardiogram (ECG), and hypertrophic or, at later stages, dilated cardiomyopathy on echocardiography. Additionally, diabetes mellitus affects 10 to 30% of FA patients.

There are atypical phenotypes with late onset presentation after the age of 25 years, which are commonly characterized by leg spasticity, retained tendon reflexes, and mild cerebellar vermian atrophy.

The patient under discussion was admitted to the neuropediatric ward. Hyperglycemia was normalized by subcutaneous administration of insulin. Additional investigations showed mild spinal cord atrophy in the cervical region on MRI, sensory neuropathy, and mild hypertrophic cardiomyopathy. Genetic testing was performed, revealing an increased number of GAA repeats (180; normal <40) within the first intron of the *frataxin* gene on chromosome 9q13, confirming the diagnosis of FA.

Genetics of Friedreich Ataxia

An increased number of GAA repeats in the *frataxin* gene is found in 98% of FA patients. There is a correlation of onset age, disease severity, and associated systemic symptoms with the repeat expansion size, which can range from 70–90 to over 1,000. About 2% of cases of FA are due to a combination of an intron 1 GAA expansion and a point mutation or deletion in the *frataxin* gene. The latter should be considered in patients with a typical clinical picture without genetic confirmation of the diagnosis, because routine genetic testing may only screen for repeat expansions. Therefore, point mutations or deletions may be overlooked. Some point mutations result in a more severe phenotype, others in a milder phenotype.

Differential Diagnosis

Several autosomal recessive ataxias without cerebellar atrophy can mimic FA. Ataxia with vitamin E deficiency typically starts before 20 years of age and head titubation can be prominent. Visual loss caused by retinitis pigmentosa is an early symptom. Compared to FA, cardiomyopathy is less common and the clinical course is more benign. The disease is caused by mutations in the gene coding the α-tocopherol transfer protein on chromosome 8q13. Vitamin E supplementation can halt disease progression and improve ataxia.

Abetalipoproteinaemia is caused by mutations in the gene for the large subunit of microsomal triglyceride transfer protein, located on chromosome 4q22–24. This protein has a role in the assembly of apolipoprotein-B containing very low density lipoproteins and chylomicrons. Onset is in the second decade with a phenotype similar to FA. Distinguishing features are lipid malabsorption, hypocholesterolaemia, acanthocytosis, and retinitis pigmentosa. Affected patients also have deficiency of lipid-soluble vitamins, particularly vitamin E. Lipid supplementation and vitamin replacement may prevent neurological complications.

Refsum disease typically starts before the age of 20 years, but sometimes much later. It is characterized by the combination of cerebellar ataxia, peripheral polyneuropathy, sensorineural deafness, retinitis pigmentosa, and anosmia. Additional clinical features include skeletal abnormalities, ichthyosis, renal failure, and cardiomyopathy. The disease is primarily caused by mutations of the gene encoding the peroxisomal enzyme phytanoyl-CoA hydroxylase on chromosome 10pter–11.2. An identical phenotype can, less commonly, be caused by mutations in the *PEX7* gene on chromosome 6q21–22.2 encoding the peroxin 7 receptor protein. Due to impaired branched-chain fatty acid α-oxidation, phytanic acid (which is present in dairy products, meat, and fish) accumulates to high levels in the body fat of affected patients, a process that is probably responsible for the clinical manifestations of the disease. Dietary restriction of phytanic acid intake helps to stop disease progression.

Other conditions that have to be considered in the differential diagnosis include ataxia with oculomotor apraxia types 1 and 2, ataxia telangiectasia, late-onset Tay-Sachs disease, ataxia due to mitochondrial DNA mutations, hereditary motor and sensory neuropathy, and hereditary spastic paraplegia. Other clinical clues usually help to distinguish these aforementioned disorders.

Treatment and Disease Course

Patients with FA should be closely followed in specialized clinics where interdisciplinary management is available. They should receive regular physiotherapy and occupational therapy, speech and orthoptic rehabilitation, psychological support, and, if necessary, orthopedic surgery for foot deformities and scoliosis. Genetic counselling by a geneticist should be provided for at-risk relatives or for parents with an affected child when parents wish to have further children. Regular cardiac assessment is mandatory including 24-hour ECG monitoring and echocardiography. Idebenone antioxidant treatment is thought to have a beneficial effect on left ventricular hypertrophy, but it is unclear whether it can prevent cardiomyopathy or halt neurological progression. Unfortunately, recent trials did not confirm previously reported neurological and cardiac benefits of idebenone.

The disease course is relentlessly progressive with increasing ataxia and weakness leading to immobility. After 20 years, most patients will be wheelchair-dependent with some degree of scoliosis. Dysphagia becomes a problem in the latter stages of the disease. Aspiration pneumonia due to dysphagia is an important cause of morbidity and mortality.

KEY POINTS TO REMEMBER ABOUT FRIEDREICH ATAXIA

- Friedreich ataxia is the most common autosomal recessive cerebellar ataxia.
- It typically commences in childhood with gait problems and progresses to involve different neurological pathways including the corticospinal and spinocerebellar tracts and sensory neurons leading to secondary dorsal column degeneration.

- Scoliosis and pes cavus are common and systemic involvement can lead to cardiomyopathy and diabetes mellitus.
- The most common mutation present in 98% of FA patients is an increased number of GAA repeats in the first intron of the *frataxin* gene on chromosome 9q13. However, in 2% of patients the disease is caused by a combination of an intron one GAA expansion and a point mutation or deletion in the *frataxin* gene.

Further Reading

Anheim, M., Tranchant, C., & Koenig, M. (2012). The autosomal recessive cerebellar ataxias. *New England Journal of Medicine, 366*, 636–646.

Ashley, C. N., Hoang, K. D., Lynch, D. R., Perlman, S. L., & Maria, B. L. (2012). Childhood ataxia: clinical features, pathogenesis, key unanswered questions, and future directions. *Journal of Child Neurology, 27*, 1095–1120.

Delatycki, M. B., & Corben, L. A. (2012). Clinical features of Friedreich ataxia. *Journal of Child Neurology, 27*, 1133–1137.

Fogel, B. L., & Perlman, S. (2007).Clinical features and molecular genetics of autosomal recessive cerebellar ataxias. *Lancet Neurology, 6*, 245–257.

Klockgether, T. (2011).Update on degenerative ataxias. *Current Opinions in Neurology, 24*, 339–345.

Marmolino, D. (2011). Friedreich's ataxia: Past, present and future. *Brain Research Reviews, 67*, 311–330.

Schulz, J. B., Boesch, S., Bürk, K., Dürr, A., Giunti, P., Mariotti, C.,... & Pandolfo, M. (2009). Diagnosis and treatment of Friedreich ataxia: a European perspective. *Nature Reviews Neurology, 5*, 222–234.

13 Mitochondrial Encephalomyopathy, Lactic Acidosis, and Stroke-like Episodes (MELAS) Syndrome

A 53-year-old lady is referred to your clinic with a complex neurological presentation.

She presented to her local hospital one year earlier with a speech disturbance associated with the sudden onset of a throbbing headache associated with nausea and vomiting. Cerebral magnetic resonance imaging (MRI) showed a high signal abnormality in the left temporal lobe. She was given a presumptive diagnosis of herpes simplex virus (HSV) encephalitis and treated with acyclovir, but polymerase chain-reaction testing for HSV in the cerebrospinal fluid was negative. A left temporal biopsy was performed, which showed spongiform changes with some neuronal sparing in a laminar distribution of the cerebral cortex. She was discharged from hospital and her speech slowly improved and eventually she was able to return to work.

Just one month prior to this appointment at your clinic, she was readmitted to hospital with a change in behavior. She became more forgetful, irritable, and easily frustrated. This was associated with frontal headaches, which were again throbbing in nature. Her husband noticed that she was acting strangely. For example, she would pick up the phone and start talking when there was nobody on the other end of the line. During her hospital admission it was noted that she had bilateral hearing loss, ptosis, and proximal muscle weakness. She also had myoclonic jerks of the left arm, although there were no changes to correlate with this clinical finding on electroencephalogram. Repeat MRI brain revealed evidence of right temporal lobe high signal intensity with a lactate peak on magnetic resonance spectroscopy (MRS). A muscle biopsy showed evidence of ragged red fibers (Figure 13-1).

Serum lactate was initially normal but was mildly elevated on follow-up (2.56 mmol/L, range 0.50 to 2.30).

On further questioning, it is evident that the patient has a long history of hearing loss. She could not remember when this first started but recalled having an abnormal audiogram in her mid-40s. This affected the higher frequencies more than the lower frequencies and required the use of a hearing aid. She also has a long history of migraine-type headaches.

There is no family history of stroke, epilepsy, hearing loss, or diabetes mellitus.

On examination, a cognitive deficit was apparent with decreased attention and concentration. Other important findings included mild ptosis bilaterally, full extra-ocular eye movements, proximal muscle weakness of the limbs with preserved reflexes and downgoing plantar responses.

What do you do now?

The diagnosis of mitochondrial encephalomyopathy, lactic acidosis, and stroke-like episodes (MELAS) syndrome is suspected. Previous reports have suggested the following three criteria for the diagnosis of MELAS: (1) stroke-like episode before 40 years of age; (2) encephalopathy characterized by seizures, dementia, or both; and (3) lactic acidosis, ragged-red fibers, or both (Hirano et al., 1992). It has been suggested that the diagnosis can considered secure if there are also at least two of the following: normal early development, recurrent headache, or recurrent vomiting. Other frequent manifestations include limb weakness, short stature, and hearing loss (Hirano & Pavlakis, 1994).

Stroke-like episodes in MELAS often manifest as transient hemiparesis or cortical blindness. Migraine headaches may become more severe during the acute phase of the stroke. Strokes may also be associated with nausea, vomiting, and seizures. The stroke-like episodes have a characteristic

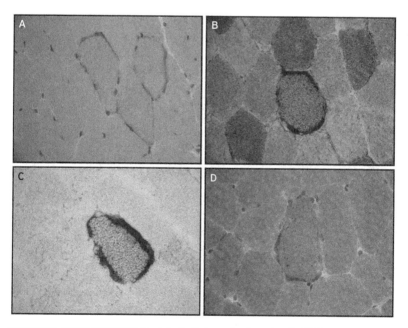

FIGURE 13-1 Muscle biopsy from the patient with haematoxylin and eosin (H&E, panel A), nicotinamide adenine dinucleotide (NADH, panel B), succinate dehydrogenase (SDH, panel C) and modified Gomori-Trichrome (panel D) staining. Ragged-red fibers were seen on Gomori-Trichrome staining (see the staining at the periphery of the muscle fiber, center of panel D).

appearance on brain MRI with areas of increased T2 signal, which often involve the posterior cerebrum and do not conform to the distribution of major arteries (an example is shown in Figure 13-2; DiMauro & Hirano, 1993; Sue, Crimmins, et al., 1998). Diffusion-weighted MRI often shows increased apparent diffusion coefficient (ADC) in the stroke-like lesions of MELAS, in contrast to the decreased ADC usually seen in ischemic strokes. Magnetic resonance spectroscopy may also be helpful, showing the presence of a lactate peak within the stroke lesion.

Individuals with MELAS are susceptible to sensorineural hearing loss that is usually gradual in onset, symmetrical, and initially affecting the higher frequencies. The hearing loss has a cochlear origin, and cochlear implantation may restore good functional hearing (Sue, Lipsett, et al., 1998).

Other clinical features that were reported to occur in a minority of patients with MELAS include diabetes mellitus, myoclonus, cerebellar signs, peripheral neuropathy, ophthalmoplegia, optic atrophy, nephropathy, cardiomyopathy, Wolff-Parkinson White syndrome, and cutaneous purpura (Hirano & Pavlakis, 1994).

The diagnosis of MELAS is based upon the clinical presentation and molecular genetic testing. The most common mutation, found in

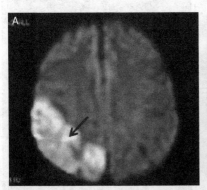 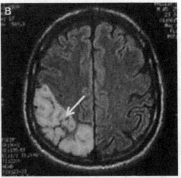

FIGURE 13-2 Typical findings on brain MRI during an acute stroke-like episode in a patient with MELAS. A. Diffusion-weighted images show increased signal in the posterior cerebrum, not conforming to either the middle or posterior cerebral artery territories (black arrow). B. T2-weighted MRI image of the same lesion (white arrow) indicating high signal predominantly involving the cerebral cortex with gyral swelling and mass effect. Adapted from a figure by Davis & Sue, with permission.

approximately 1 in 500 individuals and 80% of patients with a classical phenotype, is the m.3243A>G mutation in the *MT-TL1* gene (Manwaring et al., 2007). Other mutations in *MT-TL1*, as well as mutations in other mitochondrial DNA (mtDNA) genes such as *MT-ND5*, can also cause this disorder. Although mutations can be detected in mtDNA from leukocytes of affected individuals, the occurrence of "heteroplasmy" in disorders of mtDNA can result in variable tissue distribution of mutated mtDNA. This means that the pathogenic mutation may be undetectable in mtDNA from leukocytes and may only be detected in other tissues, such as cultured skin fibroblasts, hair follicles, urinary sediment, or skeletal muscle (Sue, Quigley, et al., 1998).

The patient had many features that were suspicious for MELAS including worsening of migrainous headaches and the occurrence of myoclonic jerks during the stroke episodes. It is not uncommon for the family history to be negative; in fact it is rare for two family members to have the full MELAS syndrome. The diagnosis of MELAS was confirmed in this patient by the identification of the m.3243A>G mutation on testing of hair follicle and muscle biopsy samples.

It is important to treat the clinical manifestations of MELAS. For example, seizures should be treated with anticonvulsant drugs, although sodium valproate should be avoided since it may increase seizure frequency in this disease (Lin & Thajeb, 2007). Other mitochondrial toxins should be avoided such as aminoglycoside antibiotics. For prevention of the primary manifestations, the administration of coenzyme Q_{10} (CoQ_{10}) and L-carnitine or idebenone (an analog of CoQ_{10}) is thought to be beneficial in some individuals. Oral administration of L-arginine appears to improve stroke-like symptoms when administered in the acute phase (within 30 minutes of stroke; Koga et al., 2005), and may reduce the frequency of strokes when given interictally, but further studies are warranted to confirm these findings.

The patient from the clinical vignette received supportive management including anticonvulsant drugs, and remains clinically stable.

KEY POINTS TO REMEMBER ABOUT MELAS SYNDROME

- Key features of mitochondrial encephalomyopathy, lactic acidosis, and stroke-like episodes (MELAS) syndrome include; stroke-like episode before 40 years of age, encephalopathy, lactic acidosis, ragged-red fibers, recurrent headache and recurrent vomiting.
- Stroke-like episodes in MELAS often manifest as transient hemiparesis or cortical blindness and can be accompanied by worsening migrainous headaches, nausea, vomiting, or seizures.
- The stroke-like episodes have a characteristic appearance on brain MRI with areas of increased T2 signal, with an increased apparent diffusion coefficient, often involving the posterior cerebrum and not conforming to the distribution of major arteries.
- The most common mutation, found in approximately 80% of individuals with a classical phenotype, is the m.3243A>G mutation in the *MT-TL1* gene.
- Coenzyme Q_{10} or idebenone may be beneficial in some individuals and L-arginine has shown promise for the treatment of acute stroke-like episodes.

Further Reading

Davis, R. L., & Sue, C. M. The genetics of mitochondrial disease. *Seminars in Neurology, 31,* 519–530.

DiMauro, S., & Hirano, M. Melas. (1993). In R. A. Pagon, M. P. Adam, T. D. Bird, TD, et al. (Eds.) *GeneReviews.* Seattle, WA: University of Washington.

Hirano, M., & Pavlakis, S. G. (1994). Mitochondrial myopathy, encephalopathy, lactic acidosis, and strokelike episodes (MELAS): Current concepts. *Journal of Child Neurology, 9,* 4–13.

Hirano, M., Ricci, E., Koenigsberger, M. R., Defindini, R., Pavlakis, S.G., DeVivo, D. C.,...& Rowland, L. P. (1992). MELAS: An original case and clinical criteria for diagnosis. *Neuromuscular Disorders, 2,* 125–135.

Koga, Y., Akita, Y., Nishioka, J., Yatsuga, S., Povalko, N., Tanabe, Y.,...& Matsuishi, T. (2005). L-arginine improves the symptoms of strokelike episodes in MELAS. *Neurology, 64,* 710–712.

Lin, C. M., & Thajeb, P. (2007). Valproic acid aggravates epilepsy due to MELAS in a patient with an A3243G mutation of mitochondrial DNA. *Metabolic Brain Disease, 22,* 105–109.

Manwaring, N., Jones, M. M., Wang, J. J., Rochtchina, E., Howard, C., Mitchell, P., & Sue, C. M. (2007). Population prevalence of the MELAS A3243G mutation. *Mitochondrion*, *7*, 230–233.

Sue, C. M., Crimmins, D. S., Soo, Y. S., Pamphlett, R., Presgrave, C. M., Kotsimbos, N., . . . & Morris, J. G. (1998). Neuroradiological features of six kindreds with MELAS tRNA(Leu) A2343G point mutation: implications for pathogenesis. *Journal of Neurology, Neurosurgery, and Psychiatry*, *65*, 233–240.

Sue, C. M., Lipsett, L. J., Crimmins, D. S., Tsang C. S., Boyages, S. C., Presgrave, C. M., . . . & Morris, J. G. (1998). Cochlear origin of hearing loss in MELAS syndrome. *Annals of Neurology*, *43*, 350–359.

Sue, C. M., Quigley, A., Katsabanis, S., Kapsa, R., Crimmins, D. S., Byrne, E., & Morris, J. G. (1998). Detection of MELAS A3243G point mutation in muscle, blood and hair follicles. *Journal of the Neurological Sciences*, *161*, 36–39.

14 Myoclonus Epilepsy and Ragged Red Fiber (MERRF)

A 43-year-old man is brought into the hospital because of an episode of sudden loss of consciousness accompanied by muscle jerking and prolonged disorientation. His brother who witnessed the episode reports that he saw the patient suddenly becoming pale and stiff with shaking all over his body while being completely unresponsive. He confirms that his brother's eyes were wide open and the color of his skin turned slightly blue before the attack stopped. It took his brother some 15 minutes until he was completely "with it" again. He has not had similar attacks before. The patient reports that he has become slightly unsteady on his feet over the last couple of years, has developed difficulties with concentration, and is bothered by occasional muscle jerking, particularly during goal-directed voluntary movements. This has frequently caused spilling of drinks. He has also noted increasing hearing problems. There is no other past medical history of note.

On neurological examination, he is fully oriented, but his report is long-winded, he is easily distractible and his thinking is generally slow. Upward gaze is slightly limited and both horizontal and vertical saccades are slow and hypometric. During testing of reflexive vertical eye movements, restricted upward gaze cannot be overcome. Fixation suppression of the vestibular-ocular reflex (VOR) is impaired. His hearing is also impaired. There is wasting of temporal and masseter muscles and weakness of shoulder, neck, and proximal leg muscles with reflexes being preserved. Arm and leg movements are dysmetric, and there is dysdiadochokinesia in the arms. His gait is wide-based ataxic, and postural stability is impaired. His speech is dysarthric. When holding out the arms and, increasingly, when reaching a target there are brief muscle jerks over and above the dysmetria.

What do you do now?

The most likely reason for the patient's admission was an epileptic seizure. Apparently, it was his first. But you suspect that this is not the typical scenario of a patient who presents with their first seizure without other medical problems. This is the story of a patient with a longer history of progressive ataxia, cognitive impairment, myopathy, mild external ophthalmoplegia, and jerky movements. Further differential diagnostic thinking hinges on the nature of the jerky movements. Jerky movements are encountered frequently in neurological practice and can cause great confusion if not accurately defined. Just as it is important to precisely distinguish between myopathic and motor-neuronal weakness, it is crucial to differentiate between tremor, chorea, and myoclonus, a task that can be challenging.

The patient's jerks were brief, nonrhythmic (unlike tremor), and not flowing or continuous (unlike chorea). To confirm your clinical suspicion of myoclonus, surface poly-electromyography (sEMG) of clinically affected muscles was performed. Results are shown in Figure 14-1.

The sEMG shows irregular jerks in biceps and triceps muscles lasting 50 milliseconds or less. On the basis of these EMG recordings alone, a definite statement about whether this is fast chorea or myoclonus cannot be made with certainty. However, the clinical presentation along with these polymyographic results makes it very likely that this is myoclonus.

Clinical re-examination shows that similar jerks are also present in leg and trunk muscles, are partly stimulus sensitive upon touch but are more

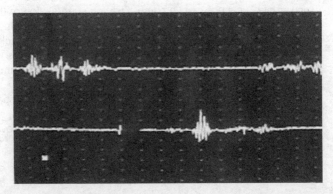

FIGURE 14-1 Surface EMG recordings from biceps (upper trace) and triceps muscle (lower trace) are shown. One division represents 50 milliseconds (ms). Irregular muscle bursts can be seen, with a duration of 50 ms or less.

likely to occur during attempted voluntary action. This clinical sign can thus be labeled as stimulus- and action-sensitive generalized myoclonus.

Such myoclonus is an important clinical clue. There are a number of conditions in which myoclonus is part of the clinical presentation, many of which have an ominous prognosis, such as Creutzfeldt-Jakob disease and subacute sclerosing panencephalitis (SSPE). The list of possible infectious, metabolic or degenerative conditions with myoclonus as a possible sign is long. However, the case under discussion has additional helpful symptoms and signs, that is, ataxia, epileptic seizures, and a myopathy including the involvement of the extra-ocular muscles.

Thus, the clinical phenotype can be summarized as a progressive myoclonus-ataxia epilepsy syndrome with an additional myopathy. A limited number of diseases are subsumed under this umbrella including Lafora body disease, neuronal ceroid lipofuscinosis, Unverricht-Lundborg disease, sialidosis, mitochondrial encephalopathies, and some disorders with spinocerebellar degeneration.

Lafora body disease is an autosomal recessive disorder characterized by periodic acid–Schiff (PAS) positive inclusions in cells of the brain, liver, muscle, and skin (particularly eccrine sweat glands). Onset is usually in childhood, with behavioral changes, cognitive decline, visual hallucinations, generalized or occipital lobe seizures, prominent photosensitivity, and myoclonus. It is caused by mutations in the gene encoding the protein laforin (epilepsy, progressive myoclonic type 2A or EPM2A) in about 75% of patients. In most other cases, mutations are found in the gene that encodes malin (also called EPM2B), a putative E3 ubiquitin ligase.

Neuronal ceroid lipofuscinosis is an autosomal recessive condition presenting with seizures, myoclonus, and dementia along with blindness in the late infantile and juvenile forms. The adult form is often dominated by behavioral changes and cognitive impairment. Lipopigment accumulates in lysosomes in the brain, eccrine glands, skin, muscle, and gut with characteristic inclusions (curvilinear bodies and fingerprint profiles). Both Lafora body disease and neuronal ceroid lipofuscinosis can usually be diagnosed on electron microscopy of axillary skin biopsies.

Unverricht-Lundborg disease (EPM1) is one of the most common progressive myoclonic encephalopathies occurring worldwide. It is inherited as an autosomal recessive trait with onset between 6 and 15 years of age and is characterized by a progressive clinical course with stimulus-sensitive myoclonus, tonic-clonic seizures, ataxia, and typical findings on EEG (such as paroxysmal generalized spike-wave activity and photosensitivity). Seizures tend to decrease in frequency in late teenage years, and cognitive function is relatively preserved. The disease is caused by mutations in the gene coding for the protein cystatin B, a member of a superfamily of cysteine protease inhibitors.

Sialidosis is also inherited as an autosomal recessive condition with onset in childhood or adolescence. The sialidoses are lysosomal storage disorders associated with a deficiency of α-N-acetylneuraminidase and, in some, with additional deficiency of alpha-galactosidase. Myoclonus in sialidosis is typically induced by action but not by light or sound. On fundoscopy, affected patients have a cherry-red spot on the retina (see chapter 11, this volume).

Mitochondrial encephalopathies can present in many different ways with a wide range for age at onset. One phenotype is the myoclonus epilepsy and ragged red fibers (MERRF) syndrome. Symptoms typically commence in the second decade, but onset can be as late as in the forties. Myoclonus and ataxia are characteristic and often presenting features. Patients also often have generalized seizures and decline cognitively in the course of the disease. Muscle weakness is variable and muscle biopsy often, but not always, shows characteristic "ragged-red" fibers (Figure 14-2).

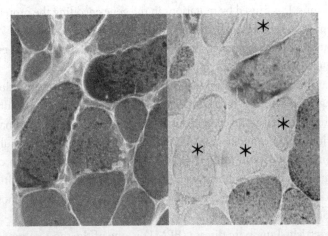

FIGURE 14-2 Muscle biopsy of a patient with MERRF. The left panel shows ragged-red fibers (modified Gomori-Trichrome staining), the right cytochrome –c oxidase negative muscle fibers (*) on cytochrome –c oxidase staining.

Deafness, short stature, and raised blood or cerebrospinal fluid lactate concentration are clues to the diagnosis of MERRF. Maternal inheritance can sometimes be evident, and a number of mutations in the mitochondrial genome have been identified.

Spinocerebellar degeneration in adults might also be associated with myoclonus. For instance, dentatorubro-pallidoluysian atrophy can present with myoclonus and epilepsy (Becher et al., 1997). Also, myoclonus can be present in some patients with the autosomal dominant cerebellar ataxias, for example, type 1, and is very characteristic in multiple-system atrophy, but the latter two conditions are typically not associated with epilepsy.

Very rarely, other disorders including Gaucher disease, GM2 gangliosidosis, biotin-responsive encephalopathy, neuroaxonal dystrophy, pantothenate associated neurodegeneration, action myoclonus-renal failure syndrome, celiac disease, and Whipple disease can cause the combination of ataxia, myoclonus, and epilepsy, but the clinical presentation is typically different.

In view of additional hearing problems and myopathy in the case under discussion, the most likely diagnosis is a mitochondrial disorder. In keeping with this, the patient had sensorineural hearing impairment, increased lactate concentration both in serum and cerebrospinal fluid, and an abnormal EEG showing intermittent generalized spike-wave and poly spike-wave complexes. MRI showed cerebellar atrophy and mild generalized brain atrophy.

Should a muscle biopsy be performed to confirm the diagnosis? This should be considered. However, given that the MERRF phenotype is correlated with mitochondrial DNA point mutations, genetic testing was initiated, which revealed a m.8344A>G transition, the most common mutation found in MERRF patients.

Additional investigations with a view to possible cardiac involvement were normal. However, neuropsychological testing showed quite marked frontal executive disturbances and impaired memory functions raising doubts about the patient's capabilities to continue his job as a civil servant. During his stay in the hospital he received psychosocial counseling and psychological support.

Since dexterity was impaired by action myoclonus, medical treatment was started.

Treatment of myoclonus can be difficult. Often, only a combination of different drugs sufficiently ameliorates the patient's symptoms.

Myoclonus in MERRF syndrome is often cortical in origin. Piracetam is probably the most effective medication to treat cortical myoclonus. It is well tolerated but usually high doses up to 24 g/day are needed. Alternatively, levetiracetam can be considered, although this is less effective. Again, high doses (between 2000–3000 mg/day) are often required. Clonazepam (1-6 mg/day) can also be used, but it causes sedation and patients may develop tolerance and become dependent.

The patient responded well to a combination of Levetiracetam 1,000 mg three times a day and clonazepam 0.5 mg twice daily, which significantly decreased myoclonic jerks and also led to improved hand function. He regularly returned to the movement disorder outpatient department without further deterioration in the following 4 years.

The prognosis of MERRF is variable. It can remain stable for many years, even for decades. Ultimately, though, the disease progresses, sometimes triggered by infection, other diseases, or some other physiologic stressor. Patients usually experience progressive ataxia, myopathy, or both, eventually leading to a severe impairment in mobility. Patients also frequently develop swallowing problems, probably caused by a combination of cerebellar dysfunction and myopathy, and can also become prone to infections and muscle wasting.

KEY POINTS TO REMEMBER ABOUT MERRF

- MERFF belongs to the group of progressive myoclonus-ataxia epilepsy syndromes and is typically characterized by additional hearing problems and myopathy.
- Onset age varies with some patients presenting in adolescence, others in the third or fourth decade.
- Muscle biopsy often shows ragged red fibers on Gomori-Trichrome stained sections.
- MERRF is most commonly caused by the mitochondrial m.8344A>G mutation.
- Treatment of myoclonus in MERRF patients can be challenging, but piracetam, levetiracetam, and clonazepam are the most effective drugs.

Further Reading

Becher, M. W., Rubinsztein, D. C., Leggo, J., Wagster, M. V., Stine, O. C., Ranen, N. G., ... & Ross, C. A. (1997). Dentatorubral and pallidoluysian atrophy (DRPLA). Clinical and neuropathological findings in genetically confirmed North American and European pedigrees. *Movement Disorders, 12,* 519–530.

Berkovic, S. F., & Andermann, F. (1986). The progressive myoclonic epilepsies. In T. A. Pedley & B. S. Meldrum (Eds.), *Recent advances in epilepsy 3* (pp.157–187). Edinburgh, Scotland: Churchill Livingstone, 1986.

Caviness, J. N., Alving, L. I., Maraganore, D. M., Black, R. A., McDonnell, S. K., & Rocca, W. A. (1999). The incidence and prevalence of myoclonus in Olmsted County, Minnesota. *Mayo Clinic Proceedings, 74,* 565–569.

Dijk, J. M., & Tijssen, M. A. J. (2010). Management of patients with myoclonus: available therapies and the need for an evidence-based approach. *Lancet Neurology, 9,* 1028–1036.

DiMauro, S., & Hirano, M. MERRF. (2009). In R. A. Pagon, T. D. Bird, C. R. Dolan et al, (Eds.) *GeneReviews.* Seattle, WA: University of Washington. Posted June 3, 2003. Updated August 18, 2009.

Gerschlager, W., & Brown, P. (2009). Myoclonus. *Current Opinions in Neurology, 22,* 414–418.

Mancuso, M., Orsucci, D., Angelini, C., Bertini, E., Carelli, V., Comi, G. P., ... & Siciliano, G. (2013). Phenotypic heterogeneity of the 8344A>G mtDNA "MERRF" mutation. *Neurology, 80,* 2049–2054.

Marsden, C. D., Harding, A. E., Obeso, J. A., & Lu, C. S. (1990). Progressive myoclonic ataxia (the Ramsay Hunt syndrome). *Archives of Neurology, 47,* 1121–1125.

Obeso, J. A. (1995). Therapy of myoclonus. *Clinical Neuroscience, 3,* 253–257.

15 POLG-Related Mitochondrial Disease

A 49-year-old woman is referred to your neurogenetics clinic with a complex neurological presentation.

She was born with bilateral footdrop and was initially thought to have had polio. She went on to have further problems with her feet and had a club foot repair on the left side at the age of 9 years. Her weakness slowly progressed until her fifth decade when she required a foot reconstruction and ankle-foot orthoses for bilateral foot drop. In the last few years she has noticed that her upper limbs and hands have now become weak. She also complains of reduced sensation in a glove-and-stocking distribution. She has received a diagnosis of Charcot-Marie Tooth (CMT) disease in the past, however, her neurologist started to question this diagnosis. In addition to distal weakness, it was observed that the patient has considerable weakness of proximal muscle groups including the neck and hip flexors. Over the past eight years she has developed severe bilateral ptosis, requiring corrective surgery six years ago. She has also noticed difficulty with swallowing. She has been seen by a gastroenterologist for constipation and transit studies demonstrated slow colonic transit but normal gastric emptying. No other family members have neurological complaints.

On clinical examination the patient has impaired visual acuity (6/12 on the right, 6/9 on the left), with bilateral optic disc pallor and retinal pigmentary change on fundoscopic examination. She had marked bilateral ptosis with impairment of upgaze. Her facial strength was preserved but she had weakness of neck flexion, neck extension and the sternocleidomastoids bilaterally. Upper limb examination revealed normal tone, diffuse weakness, areflexia, and mild intention tremor with dysdiadochokinesis. Lower limb examination revealed normal tone, and both proximal and distal weakness with foot drop and areflexia. There was distal impairment of all sensory modalities in a glove-and-stocking distribution. Gait examination revealed a high-stepping gait with sensory ataxia.

What do you do now?

You agree with the referring clinician that the diagnosis of CMT should be questioned. In particular, the presence of ptosis and ophthalmoplegia raise the possibility of mitochondrial disease.

You arrange several investigations, including nerve conduction studies, which show evidence of a generalized axonal sensorimotor polyneuropathy. Needle electromyography reveals evidence of chronic denervation. You also order brain magnetic resonance imaging (MRI) and magnetic resonance spectroscopy (MRS). Brain MRI reveals white matter hyperintensities that were more than expected for her age, and MRS did not demonstrate an elevated lactate peak. Her serum creatinine kinase is mildly elevated at 637 U/L (range 30-190). Cardiac investigations including electrocardiogram, Holter monitor, and transthoracic echocardiogram were unremarkable.

A skeletal muscle biopsy is ordered, which demonstrated features of a neuropathic process coupled with light microscopic evidence of a mitochondrial myopathy, including occasional ragged red fibers and succinic dehydrogenase positive/cytochrome c oxidase negative fibers. There were also ultrastructural changes of a mitochondrial myopathy on electron microscopy.

The biopsy appears to confirm your suspicion that the patient has a form of mitochondrial disease. It is notable that in addition to her other neurological manifestations, the patient has a progressive external ophthalmoplegia (PEO) phenotype. Progressive external ophthalmoplegia is characterized by ptosis, which is usually but not always symmetrical, accompanied by a progressive limitation of eye movements and preservation of pupillary function. Sporadic PEO and sporadic Kearns-Sayre syndrome are the most common forms and are usually due to mitochondrial DNA (mtDNA) deletions. Features of Kearns-Sayre syndrome include PEO, pigmentary retinopathy, elevated protein in the cerebrospinal fluid (CSF), cerebellar ataxia, and heart block, with onset before 20 years of age (Davis & Sue, 2011; DiMauro & Hirano, 1993). The PEO phenotype can be maternally inherited due to mtDNA point mutations (including the MELAS m.A3243G mutation). Several nuclear-encoded genes can also cause a PEO phenotype, including: (a) *SLC25A4*, encoding the ANT1 protein, (b) *C10orf2* (previously known as *PEO1*), encoding the Twinkle protein, (c) *POLG* encoding DNA polymerase subunit gamma, (d) *TYMP*, encoding thymidine phosphorylase, (e) and *OPA1* encoding the OPA1 protein (DiMauro & Hirano, 1993). Other disorders can cause a PEO-like phenotype (e.g. myasthenia gravis, oculopharyngeal muscular dystrophy, oculopharyngodistal myopathy, myotonic dystrophy type 1, and myopathy caused by mutations in *MYH2*) but are much less likely in this case.

Urine purines and pyrimidines were ordered but did not show any evidence of MNGIE syndrome (which is caused by *TYMP* mutations, see chapter 16, this volume). You also consider performing a lumbar puncture in order to determine whether there is increased protein in the CSF. Another option would be to request a Southern blot analysis of muscle mtDNA in order to investigate for mtDNA deletions. However, in the first instance, the patient was enrolled in a study in which patients were screened for mutations in the *POLG* gene (Woodbridge, Liang, Davis, Vandebona, & Sue, 2013). This revealed that she was a compound heterozygote for *POLG* mutations (p.T851A and p.N468D), consistent with the diagnosis of POLG-related mitochondrial disease.

Mutations in *POLG* gene, the gene encoding the only mtDNA polymerase, are, by far, the commonest cause of mtDNA stability disorders (Chinnery & Hudson, 2013). Mutations in this gene can cause either point mutations (through impaired mtDNA proofreading) or deletions (through disturbed polymerase activity) in mtDNA. Conditions related to *POLG* mutations can be inherited as either autosomal recessive or autosomal dominant traits. Clinical features may include PEO, ataxia, peripheral neuropathy, seizures, gastrointestinal symptoms, parkinsonism, and psychiatric disturbance. Moreover, children may present with Alpers syndrome or hepatocerebral disease associated with mtDNA depletion. Care must be taken to avoid treatment with sodium valproate, which may potentially exacerbate seizures and hepatic impairment.

You continue to see the patient in the neurogenetics clinic and arrange for ongoing physiotherapy, occupational therapy, and speech pathology input. You also start her on coenzyme Q10 supplementation, since this is a candidate therapy for mtDNA depletion syndromes (Montero et al., 2013).

Further Reading

Chinnery, P. F., & Hudson, G. (2013). Mitochondrial genetics. *British Medical Bulletin, 106,* 135–159.

Davis, R. L., & Sue, C. M. (2011). The genetics of mitochondrial disease. *Seminars in Neurology, 31,* 519–530.

DiMauro, S., & Hirano, M. (1993). Mitochondrial DNA deletion syndromes. In: R. A. Pagon, M. P. Adam, T. D. Bird, C. R. Dolan, C. T. Fong, K. Stephens (Eds.). *GeneReviews.* Seattle, WA: University of Washington.

Montero, R., Grazina, M., López-Gallardo, E., Montoya, J., Briones, P., Navarro-Sastre, A.,... & Artuch, R. (2013). Coenzyme Q10 deficiency in mitochondrial DNA depletion syndromes. *Mitochondrion, 13,* 337–341.

Woodbridge, P., Liang, C., Davis, R. L., Vandebona, H., & Sue, C. M. (2013). POLG mutations in Australian patients with mitochondrial disease. *Internal Medicine Journal, 43,* 150–156.

16 Mitochondrial Neurogastrointestinal Encephalopathy (MNGIE) Syndrome

A 38-year-old man presents to your clinic after more than 10 years of neurological symptoms (as we have previously reported; Needham, Duley, Hammond, Herkes, Hirano, & Sue, 2007).

He first noticed symptoms from the age of 27 years, with cramping and pain in his legs while working as a hairdresser. There were no associated sensory symptoms.

Nerve conduction studies performed at the time of presentation were thought to be consistent with a demyelinating rather than axonal peripheral neuropathy (Table 16-1).

The patient was diagnosed with Charcot-Marie-Tooth (CMT) disease according to the clinical and neurophysiological findings, but this diagnosis was not confirmed with genetic testing.

At the age of 35 years, the patient began to develop cramping abdominal pain associated with a decrease in appetite, early satiety, and marked weight loss. He recalled having prominent "tummy rumbles" (borborygmi) throughout childhood. On examination he was markedly cachectic. He had wasting in the facial muscles, shoulder girdle, and distal extremities. He also had a complex external ophthalmoplegia with bilateral ptosis, as well as facial and limb muscle weakness, absent deep tendon reflexes in the lower limbs, and bilateral pes cavus with clawed toes.

While in the clinic, a detailed family history is taken. The patient is the third of four male siblings, and his parents are first cousins (Figure 16-1). The patient mentions that his second eldest brother died at the age of 29 years from a "ruptured diverticulum," and so with permission the brother's clinical notes were reviewed.

The patient's brother (II.2) was diagnosed with noninsulin dependent diabetes mellitus at the age of 24 years. At the age of 28 years he underwent a resection of his appendix and was found to have a small congenital intestinal (Meckel) diverticulum. Following this, he had recurrent abdominal abscesses, a spontaneous small bowel perforation and bilateral pneumonia. He died shortly afterward from a cardiopulmonary arrest and sepsis. An autopsy was not performed. While in the hospital, he was noted to have a peripheral neuropathy with weak ankle movements, reduced deep tendon reflexes, a complex external ophthalmoplegia, bilateral ptosis, and reduced gastrointestinal (GI) motility.

What do you do now?

The clinical presentation is strongly suspicious of a condition known as MNGIE syndrome (*mitochondrial, neurogastrointestinal encephalopathy*). This is a rare autosomal recessive condition due to mutations in the *thymidine phosphorylase* (*TYMP*) gene. This gene encodes the enzyme thymidine phosphorylase, which catalyses the conversion of thymidine to thymine. Most mutations markedly reduce or abolish activity of this enzyme, which results in raised levels of thymidine.

The clinical features of MNGIE include (a) GI dysmotility; (b) cachexia; (c) ptosis, ophthalmoparesis, or both; (d) peripheral neuropathy; and (e) leukoencephalopathy (Hirano, Nishigaki, & Marti, 2004). The average age at onset is about 19 years old but varies from 5 months to 43 years. Gastrointestinal dysmotility can involve any section of the enteric system from the oropharynx to the small intestine. The specific manifestations include borborygmi, diarrhea, early satiety, nausea, vomiting, abdominal cramping, intestinal pseudo-obstruction and gastroparesis. Cachexia is a striking feature in all MNGIE patients and is partly attributable to GI

TABLE 16-1 **Nerve conduction studies in the proband suggesting a demyelinating peripheral neuropathy**

	Latency	Amplitude	Conduction velocity
Motor nerve conduction studies			
Peroneal Nerve: ankle to EDB	7	1.6	
Peroneal Nerve: knee to EDB		0.5	27
Tibial nerve: ankle to AH	7.3	2.2	
Tibial nerve: knee to AH		1.9	25
Median nerve: wrist to APB	5.7	5.6	
Median nerve: elbow to APB		3.7	32
Sensory nerve conduction studies			
Sural	Absent		
Median nerve: wrist to index	5.2	13	
Median nerve: elbow to index	10.4	3	42

AH, abductor hallicus; APB, abductor pollicis brevis; EDB, extensor digitorum brevis.

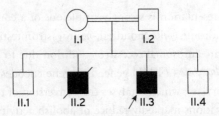

FIGURE 16-1 Pedigree of family with neurological and gastrointestinal symptoms. Males are represented by squares, females by circles. A diagonal line through the symbol indicates a deceased individual. Filled symbols indicate affected family members. The index patient (II.3) is indicated with an arrow. A consanguineous relationship is represented by a double horizontal line.

dysfunction (Hirano et al., 2004). In contrast to the GI symptoms, the neurological symptoms of peripheral neuropathy, ptosis, ophthalmoparesis, and hearing loss are relatively mild.

The patient described in the clinical vignette had many clinical features that were distinctive for MNGIE syndrome such as GI dysmotility, cachexia, ptosis, ophthalmoparesis, and peripheral neuropathy. The family history of consanguinity is suggestive of an autosomal recessive disorder due to homozygous mutations. It is not uncommon for patients with MNGIE to be misdiagnosed as having CMT (Needham et al., 2007; Said et al., 2005), as occurred in the proband (II.3). It is also notable that small intestinal dysmotility leads to a high frequency of diverticula in the duodenum and jejunum of patients with MNGIE. In some patients with MNGIE, this can be complicated by rupture of the diverticula resulting in fatal peritonitis, and it is likely that this scenario occurred in the proband's brother (II.2).

In order to investigate for gastrointestinal dysmotility, the patient had a whole GI scintigraphy study that revealed markedly abnormal gastric emptying but normal colonic transit.

You also order a cerebral MRI that revealed evidence of widespread generalized increased signal intensity on T2 weighting throughout the deep white matter and extending into the brainstem, consistent with a leukoencephalopathy (Figure 16-2).

He was also found to have low thymidine phosphorylase activity in the buffy coat, associated with an increased concentration of plasma thymidine and deoxyuridine. DNA sequencing showed a homozygotic 20 base-pair

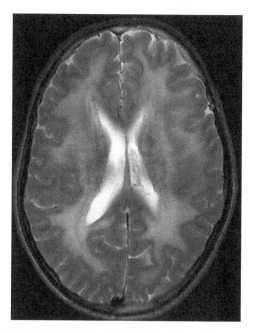

FIGURE 16-2 Axial T2 weighted MRI in the patient showing evidence of widespread generalized increased signal intensity throughout the white matter.

deletion in exon 10 of the *TYMP* gene, thus confirming the diagnosis of MNGIE syndrome.

Supportive measures are the mainstay of treatment for MNGIE. For the treatment of abdominal cramps, it may be useful to assess the patient for intestinal bacterial overgrowth (e.g., using a hydrogen breath test). If the breath test is positive, the patient may require treatment with antibiotics. Treatment for dysmotility can be attempted with stool softeners (as long as the patient does not have diarrhea), or drugs to increase bowel motility. However, affected patients will usually have degeneration of the intestinal smooth muscle, so treatment of this manifestation is unlikely to be effective.

Patients with MNGIE will often become severely cachexic, and so efforts to maintain their nutritional status are vital. Their diet should be carefully monitored and include the appropriate vitamin supplements such as iron, calcium, and vitamin D. Sufferers may require feeding via percutaneous gastrostomy (PEG). Intravenous nutritional support using total parenteral nutrition (TPN) can also be used to temporarily help some patients by bypassing the GI tract (Hirano et al., 2004).

Allogeneic hematopoietic stem cell transplant has been proposed as a treatment for patients with MNGIE with a view to restoring thymidine phosphorylase activity, and standardised transplant protocols have recently been published (Halter et al., 2011).

The prognosis of MNGIE is poor, with many patients dying at an early age (Hirano et al., 2004). The patient from the clinical vignette has struggled to maintain his weight and suffers from ongoing anorexia, fatigue and postprandial abdominal spasms. He was managed with dietician and speech therapy input and medical therapy with domperidone, coenzyme Q10, magnesium, vitamin D, iron, proton pump inhibitors and laxatives. He received a course of treatment with cephalexin for presumed small bowel bacterial overgrowth. He refused PEG feeding, nasogastric tube feeding, and TPN. He declined a bone marrow transplantation. His weight is currently stable and he continues to remain relatively active and independent at the age of 47 years.

KEY POINTS TO REMEMBER ABOUT MNGIE SYNDROME

- The clinical features of MNGIE (mitochondrial, neurogastrointestinal encephalopathy) syndrome include GI dysmotility, cachexia, ptosis, ophthalmoparesis, peripheral neuropathy, and leukoencephalopathy.
- MNGIE can present with a phenotype resembling Charcot-Marie-Tooth Disease.
- Laboratory assessment of thymidine phosphorylase enzyme activity can be useful.
- Genetic testing for mutations in the *thymidine phosphorylase* (*TYMP*) gene can confirm the diagnosis.
- Treatment consists of supportive measures such as maintaining the patient's nutritional status; the patient may also be a candidate for an allogeneic hematopoietic stem cell transplant.

Further Reading

Halter, J., Schüpbach, W. M., Casali, C., Elhasid, R., Fay, K., Hammans, S.,... & Hirano, M. (2011). Allogeneic hematopoietic SCT as treatment option for patients with mitochondrial neurogastrointestinal encephalomyopathy (MNGIE): a consensus conference proposal for a standardized approach. *Bone Marrow Transplantation, 46,* 330–337.

Hirano, M., Nishigaki, Y., & Marti, R. (2004). Mitochondrial neurogastrointestinal encephalomyopathy (MNGIE): a disease of two genomes. *The Neurologist, 10,* 8–17.

Needham, M., Duley, J., Hammond, S., Herkes, G. K., Hirano, M., & Sue, C. M. (2007). Mitochondrial disease mimicking Charcot-Marie Tooth disease. *Journal of Neurology, Neurosurgery, and Psychiatry, 78,* 99–100.

Said, G., Lacroix, C., Planté-Bordeneuve, V., Messing, B., Slama, A., Crenn, P.,... & Matuchansky, C. (2005). Clinicopathological aspects of the neuropathy of neurogastrointestinal encephalomyopathy (MNGIE) in four patients including two with a Charcot-Marie-Tooth presentation. *Journal of Neurology, 252,* 655–662.

17 Leber Hereditary Optic Neuropathy

A 37-year-old woman is referred to the neurogenetics clinic for further investigations and management of her neurological condition.

Her first symptoms began at the age of 31 years, after the birth of her daughter, when she noticed paraesthesia in her right leg. At the age of 36 years she developed back pain associated with further tingling in her right leg, which was followed by paraesthesia in her left leg and anaesthesia of both feet. Approximately six months later, she noticed that she was losing focus in her right eye. She was referred for a magnetic resonance imaging (MRI) scan of the brain, which showed white matter lesions indicative of demyelinating plaques, in keeping with the diagnosis of multiple sclerosis (MS). She also developed worsening gait ataxia at the time requiring admission to the local hospital. Examination of the cerebrospinal fluid (CSF) revealing oligoclonal bands, which were not present in the serum. She was subsequently treated with a course of intravenous methylprednisolone with an improvement in her neurological symptoms.

Salient findings on examination include impairment of visual acuity (right 6/24 and left 6/12) and a relative afferent pupillary defect on the right side. Fundoscopy revealed optic nerve atrophy on the right. Additional findings included corticospinal tract signs (hyperreflexia) and heel-shin ataxia in the limbs, signs of sensory impairment predominantly involving the right leg, and an ataxic gait.

Interestingly, there is a family history of Leber hereditary optic neuropathy (LHON). The patient's mother was diagnosed with LHON as well as an MS-like illness. She also had an ataxic gait. Additionally, her younger brother, maternal uncle, and maternal grandmother have also been diagnosed with LHON. Several affected family members have been genetically tested for LHON and were shown to have the m.11778G>A mutation.

What do you do now?

The patient appears to have both LHON and an MS-like illness.

Leber hereditary optic neuropathy is caused by mutations in mitochondrial DNA and is transmitted by maternal inheritance. It is characterized by bilateral, painless, subacute visual loss that usually develops in early adult life (Yu-Wai-Man & Chinnery, 1993). Males are four to five times more likely to be affected than females. Affected individuals develop monocular visual blurring affecting the central vision; often with sequential visual loss in the other eye an average of two to three months later (Davis & Sue, 2011). In approximately 25% of cases, the visual loss is bilateral at disease onset. Visual acuity is severely reduced to counting fingers or worse in most cases, and visual fielding testing demonstrates an enlarging dense central or centrocecal scotoma. Following the acute phases, the optic discs become atrophic, and loss of visual acuity is most likely permanent. Other neurological abnormalities such as peripheral neuropathy can occur.

Investigations for LHON include dilated fundoscopy in order to identify characteristic optic disc and vascular changes in the acute phase. Detailed visual field testing (e.g., Goldman visual field exam) may be useful to delineate the characteristic central or centrocecal scotoma. Electrophysiological studies may be useful such as visually evoked potentials (VEPs) to confirm optic nerve dysfunction and pattern electroretinogram to exclude retinal disease. Neuroimaging is also important to exclude compressive, infiltrative and inflammatory causes of optic atrophy. About 90% patients with LHON will have one of three point mutations in mitochondrial DNA; m.3460G>A, m.11778G>A, or m.14484T>C.

An MS-like illness occurring in women who have LHON is known as "Harding" disease (Harding et al., 1992). A recent study showed that the co-occurrence of MS and LHON mtDNA mutations is likely due to chance (Pfeffer, Burke, Yu-Wai-Man, Compston, & Chinnery, 2013). However, patients with MS and LHON had multiple episodes of visual loss, were predominantly women, and had a longer time interval before the fellow eye was affected (on average 1.66 years)—findings that are atypical of LHON. Most patients present without eye pain and have a poor visual prognosis, which is also unusual for optic neuritis associated with MS. This suggests that the co-occurrence of MS and LHON results in a disorder that has a distinct clinical phenotype.

The patient described in the clinical vignette had a homoplasmic m.117798G>A mutation on genetic analysis of her urinary cell pellet. Homoplasmy indicates all copies of mtDNA are identical, and urinary sediment is often tested because this tissue is easily obtained and can reliably detect mtDNA mutations in affected patients. Visual evoked potentials were performed and showed delayed P100 latencies for the right eye. Interestingly, a recent randomized placebo controlled trial showed that patients with LHON who had discordant visual acuities are the most likely to benefit from idebenone treatment, which is a safe and well-tolerated therapy (Klopstock et al., 2011). The patient was trialed on idebenone, but she stopped this medication after failing to notice any benefit. This patient continued to have relapses of MS (see Figure 17-1 for follow-up MRI) and was referred to the MS clinic for consideration of disease modifying therapies.

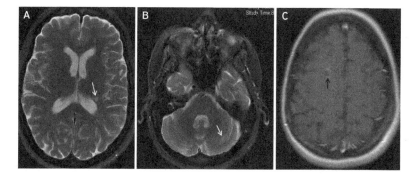

FIGURE 17-1 Follow-up MRI of the patient from the clinical vignette with Leber hereditary optic neuropathy. A. Axial T2-weighted image showing a periventricular plaque (white arrow). B. Axial T2-weighted image showing a single lesion within the left cerebellar hemisphere (white arrow). C. Axial T1-weighted image postintravenous gadolinium showing a lesion in the right frontal lobe (black arrow) with central cystic change and periventricular enhancement suggestive of an active lesion.

KEY POINTS TO REMEMBER ABOUT LEBER HEREDITARY OPTIC NEUROPATHY

- Leber hereditary optic neuropathy (LHON) is characterized by bilateral (usually sequential), painless, subacute visual loss that usually develops in early adult life.
- It affects males four to five times more frequently than females.
- About 90% patients with LHON will have one of three point mutations in mitochondrial DNA; m.3460G>A, m.11778G>A, or m.14484T>C.
- Treatment with idebenone may be beneficial.
- Co-occurrence of multiple sclerosis and LHON (known as Harding disease) appears to be coincidental but may lead to a distinctive clinical phenotype.

Further Reading

Davis, R. L., & Sue, C. M. (2011).The genetics of mitochondrial disease. *Seminars in Neurology, 31,* 519–530.

Harding, A. E., Sweeney, M. G., Miller, D. H., Mumford, C. J., Kellar-Wood, H., Menard, D.,...& Compston, D. A. (1992). Occurrence of a multiple sclerosis-like illness in women who have a Leber's hereditary optic neuropathy mitochondrial DNA mutation. *Brain: A Journal of Neurology, 115*(Pt 4), 979–989.

Klopstock, T., Yu-Wai-Man, P., Dimitriadis, K., Rouleau, J., Heck, S., Bailie, M.,...& Chinnery, P. F. (2011). A randomized placebo-controlled trial of idebenone in Leber's hereditary optic neuropathy. *Brain: A Journal of Neurology, 134,* 2677–2686.

Pfeffer, G., Burke, A., Yu-Wai-Man, P., Compston, D. A., & Chinnery, P. F. (2013). Clinical features of MS associated with Leber hereditary optic neuropathy mtDNA mutations. *Neurology, 81,* 2073–2081.

Yu-Wai-Man, P., Chinnery, P. F. (1993). Leber hereditary optic neuropathy. In. R. A. Pagon, M. P. Adam, T. D. Bird, C. R. Dolan, C. T. Fong, & K. Stephens (Eds.), *GeneReviews*. Seattle, WA: University of Washington.

18 Charcot-Marie-Tooth Disease Type 1

A 35-year-old woman is admitted to the neurology department because of a several-year history of tingling and burning in her feet, gait unsteadiness, and tripping. She first noticed problems while playing school sports in her late teens, with difficulties running fast and jumping, and a tendency to sprain her joints. Also, some of her classmates had commented on her legs resembling those of a stork with very slim calves and ankles. In her 20s she began to use orthopedic footwear that increased the stability of her walking. Her current main symptoms are unpleasant sensations in both feet as if she was walking on a hot surface. Her past medical history is unremarkable. As far as she knows no other family member is affected. She has two brothers.

On examination, close inspection and palpation reveals thickening of the greater auricular nerves and ulnar nerves at the elbow. Cranial nerves are normal. There is mild wasting of the thenar and hypothenar eminences bilaterally, thinning of both calves giving rise to an "inverted champagne" bottle appearance of her legs and marked wasting of intrinsic foot muscles with bilateral pes cavus and hammer toes. Weakness is observed in the intrinsic hand muscles (4/5), proximal leg muscles (4/5), and for ankle dorsiflexion (3/5), inversion (3/5) and eversion (2/5) as well as for toe extension (2/5). Reflexes cannot be elicited. The Babinski sign is negative bilaterally. There is decreased pin prick and touch sensation in a glove-and-stocking distribution. Using a vibration threshold scale, vibration sense is reduced to 2/8 distally at her fingers and 0/8 in the leg. When holding out the arms in front of her, mild pseudo-athetoid movements are noted. She has an unsteady, high-stepping gait.

What do you do now?

Clearly, the clinical presentation is that of a chronic motor and sensory neuropathy without signs of an involvement of other systems. Given that there is a foot deformity, a long disease process and an early disease-onset are likely, as is often the case in hereditary neuropathies. To confirm this suspicion, clinical examination of additional family members is helpful, and so a visit by one of her brothers is arranged. He does not report symptoms other than occasionally tripping. On examination, he also has slim calves, pes cavus, and marked atrophy of the intrinsic foot muscles. There is weakness of ankle dorsiflexion, tendon reflexes are abolished, and touch and vibration sensation is reduced distally. He also has a stepping gait. In old photographs taken during a summer holiday it can be confirmed that their father also had very slim legs and pes cavus. Taken together, the most likely diagnosis is autosomal dominant hereditary motor and sensory neuropathy (HMSN), also called Charcot-Marie-Tooth (CMT) disease.

Charcot Marie Tooth Disease—An Overview

CMT disease, (or HMSN), is the most common inherited disorder of the peripheral nervous system, and one of the most common groups of human hereditary disorders with a prevalence of around 1/2500. The clinical presentation is manifold with onset ranging from infancy to late adulthood. Most types of CMT are inherited in an autosomal dominant fashion (CMT type 1 and 2), but there are also X-linked (CMTX) or autosomal recessive forms. Mutations in more than 40 genes have been identified.

The clinical hallmarks are wasting and weakness of distal limb muscles, skeletal deformities including pes cavus (caused by selective denervation of intrinsic foot muscles), and reduced or absent tendon reflexes. Affected patients are liable to episodes of pressure palsies. Sensory deficits and pain are variable but can be troublesome.

The severity of CMT ranges from severe forms of demyelinating neuropathy, also called Dejerine–Sottas disease (DSD), to very mild forms without significant disability. Sensory gait ataxia is common.

The classification of HMSN is confusing and disputed. Classically, two main forms are distinguished on the basis of electrophysiological features, that is, demyelinating and axonal, with further subcategorization into seven types: HMSN type I corresponding to demyelinating forms with autosomal

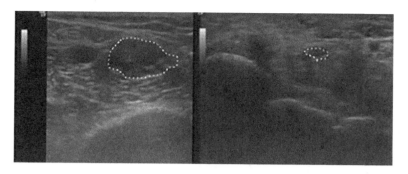

FIGURE 18-1 Ultrasound image of a median nerve section at the wrist of a patient with CMT disease type 1 (left panel) and a healthy control subject (right panel).

dominant, autosomal recessive, or X-linked inheritance; HMSN type II corresponding to axonal forms with autosomal dominant, autosomal recessive, or X-linked inheritance; HMSN type III (also referred to as DSD); HMSN type IV (Refsum disease); HMSN type V (HMSN associated with paraplegia); HMSN type VI (HMSN with optic atrophy); and HMSN type VII (HMSN with retinitis pigmentosa).

Traditionally, a cutoff of 38 meters per second (m/s) for median nerve motor conduction velocity was proposed as the key electrodiagnostic marker (values < 38 m/s being characteristic for CMT1 and > 38 m/s for CMT2).

Electrodiagnostic studies of our case showed profoundly decreased median nerve motor conduction velocity (15 m/s) bilaterally suggestive of CMT1. In keeping with the clinical finding of hypertrophic nerves, an ultrasound demonstrated markedly increased diameter of nerves and plexus fascicles including the median nerve at the wrist (Figure 18-1).

Genetic Testing in Charcot-Marie-Tooth Disease Type 1

The most common CMT1 subtype, in fact the most common of all CMT diseases, is CMT1A caused by a 17p12 duplication encompassing the coding region of the myelin protein PMP22. This duplication leads to a 50% increase in *PMP22* gene expression. It accounts for about 70% of CMT1 cases and 50% of all types of CMT [34]. It was also found in the case described here.

Other CMT1 subtypes are CMT1B caused by mutation in the *P0* gene that can lead to deafness and pupillary abnormalities in addition to polyneuropathy, CMT1C due to *LITAF* gene mutations, which are typically associated with arm tremor and gait ataxia, CMT1D on the basis of *EGR2* gene mutations where affected patients often have scoliosis, CMT1E due to *PMP22* mutations, and CMT1F due to *NEFL* gene mutations. Hearing loss can occur in the latter two subtypes.

Charcot-Marie-Tooth Disease Type 1A
CMT1A is characterized by slowly progressive distal muscle weakness and atrophy primarily affecting the small foot and peroneal muscles early in the course of the disease and the intrinsic hand and forearm muscles in the latter stages of disease. In addition, there are distal, usually symmetric sensory deficits in almost all patients and foot deformities including pes cavus and claw toes in most. Tendon reflexes are diminished or absent. Symptoms and signs progress slowly. Often, the disease is benign, and most patients do not become wheelchair dependent. Typically, there is a striking discrepancy between the marked clinical signs and relatively few or mild symptoms. Many affected relatives of patients seeking medical advice have little or no symptoms. Therefore, when a hereditary neuropathy is suspected, family members should be examined personally because verbal confirmation of the family history is unreliable.

Management
Currently, no specific treatment is available for CMT diseases. Supportive and preventive measures include regular physiotherapy, orthopedic footwear, and technical aids. Medical treatment of neuropathic pain is often helpful.

Clinical trials of products that have been shown to downregulate *PMP22* messenger RNA expression in primary cultures of rat Schwann cells are ongoing.

- CMT diseases encompass a large spectrum of hereditary neuropathies with a very diverse genetic background.
- CMT1A is the most common hereditary neuropathy and is characterized by a slowly progressive motor and sensory polyneuropathy and foot deformities.
- Electrophysiologically, CMT1A is defined by a reduced motor-nerve conduction velocity (< 38 m/s). Hypertrophic nerves can often be visualized by ultrasound.
- CMT1A is an autosomal dominant disease caused by a 17p12 duplication encompassing the *PMP22* gene.

Further Reading

Azzedine, H., Senderek, J., Rivolta, C., & Chrast, R. (2012). Molecular genetics of Charcot-Marie-Tooth disease: From genes to genomes. *Molecular Syndromology, 3*, 204–214.

Dyck, P. J., & Lambert, E. H. (1968). Lower motor and primary sensory neuron diseases with peroneal muscular atrophy. I. Neurologic, genetic, and electrophysiologic findings in hereditary polyneuropathies. *Archives of Neurology, 18*, 603–618.

Dyck, P.J., & Lambert, E. H. (1968). Lower motor and primary sensory neuron diseases with peroneal muscular atrophy. II. Neurologic, genetic, and electrophysiologic findings in various neuronal degenerations. *Archives of Neurology, 18*, 619–625.

Gallardo, E., Garcia, A., Combarros, O., & Berciano, J. (2006). Charcot-Marie-Tooth disease type 1A duplication: Spectrum of clinical and magnetic resonance imaging features in leg and foot muscles. *Brain: A Journal of Neurology, 129*, 426–437.

Murphy, S. M., Laura, M., Fawcett, K., Pandraud, A., Liu, Y. T., Davidson, G. L., ...& Reilly, M. M. (2012). Charcot-Marie-Tooth disease: frequency of genetic subtypes and guidelines for genetic testing. *Journal of Neurology, Neurosurgery, & Psychiatry, 83*, 706–710.

Verhamme, C., van Schaik, I. N., Koelman, J. H. T. M., de Haan, R. J., & de Visser, M. (2009). The natural history of Charcot–Marie-Tooth type 1A in adults: A 5-year follow-up study. *Brain: A Journal of Neurology, 132*, 3252–3262.

19 Hereditary Neuropathy with Liability to Pressure Palsies

A 58-year-old man is referred to your neurology clinic for sensory symptoms in the left leg.

He was diagnosed with polio at the age of 5 years after suffering leg weakness (he was unable to recall which leg was presumably affected). He suffered recurrence of his leg weakness at the age of 6 or 7 years, was treated with lower back surgery, and eventually his leg symptoms improved. He had a fairly normal adult life until the age of 39 years when he was diagnosed with a common peroneal nerve lesion on the left side, which was attributed to excessive leg crossing. His symptoms improved spontaneously.

Over the last few months, he has experienced further numbness and a tight sensation over his left leg. He informs you that there is a dull discomfort of the entire left leg below the knee. The symptoms were initially progressive but are now stable.

The patient also has a history of bilateral carpal tunnel syndrome, treated with nocturnal wrist splinting.

Clinical examination of the upper limbs revealed depressed deep-tendon reflexes and diminished pinprick sensation in a median nerve distribution bilaterally. There was no wasting or weakness of the thumb abductors or intrinsic muscles of the hand on either side. Lower limb examination revealed no evidence of atrophy or fasciculations, tone and power were normal, and plantars were down-going. However, the reflexes were again depressed, and there was diminished sensation to pinprick for the lateral surface of the left leg below the knee. There were no signs of cranial nerve involvement, palpable nerves, or pes cavus.

The family history reveals that his brother and his brother's daughter have had similar symptoms.

What do you do now?

You order a nerve conduction study (Figure 19-1).

The nerve conduction study has revealed several interesting findings. The motor studies for the left common peroneal nerve show slowing across the fibular head, without conduction block, which could be in keeping with a compressive lesion at this site. For the median nerve, the distal motor latencies are markedly prolonged bilaterally. In addition, the median nerve sensory studies are either very low amplitude with a slowed conduction velocity (on the right) or absent (on the left), consistent with carpal tunnel lesions at the wrists. Furthermore, the ulnar nerve motor studies show slowing of conduction velocity across both the elbows (without conduction block), consistent with mild bilateral ulnar nerve entrapments.

In this case, the diagnosis of hereditary neuropathy with liability to pressure palsies (HNPP) should be considered given that the patient has had recurrent focal compressive neuropathies and a family history consistent with autosomal dominant inheritance.

Findings that can be seen in HNPP include (a) the presence of a mild polyneuropathy (with or without symptoms), (b) evidence on physical examination of previous nerve palsies such as focal weakness, atrophy or sensory impairment, (c) the absence of ankle reflexes (50-80%), (d) a diffuse reduction in deep tendon reflexes (15-30%), and (e) a mild to moderate pes cavus foot deformity (20%). In this patient, the deep tendon reflexes are diffusely depressed, consistent with the diagnosis of HNPP (Bird, 1993).

In addition to the typical presentation, patients with HNPP can have other phenotypes such as recurrent positional short-term sensory symptoms, a progressive mononeuropathy, Charcot-Marie Tooth-like polyneuropathy, chronic sensory polyneuropathy, and a chronic inflammatory demyelinating polyneuropathy-like disorder. Some patients may also be asymptomatic.

Electrodiagnostic studies are usually abnormal in HNPP. There may be a diffuse increase in distal motor latencies contrasting with normal or moderately reduced motor nerve conduction velocities, a diffuse reduction in SNAPs, and multiple focal slowing of nerve conduction at the typical sites of entrapment. However, the key diagnostic criterion is bilateral slowing of sensory and motor median nerve conduction at the carpal tunnel with at least one abnormal parameter for motor conduction in one peroneal nerve (Mouton et al., 1999).

Motor Nerve Conduction:

Nerve and Site	Latency	Amplitude	Segment	Latency Difference	Distance	Conduction Velocity
Peroneal L						
Ankle	7.0 ms	1.3 mV	Extensor digitorum brevis-Ankle	7.0 ms	85 mm	m/s
Fibula (head)	13.5 ms	1.7 mV	Ankle-Fibula (head)	6.5 ms	300 mm	46 m/s
Popliteal fossa	16.6 ms	1.5 mV	Fibula (head)-Popliteal fossa	3.1 ms	85 mm	27 m/s
Tibial L						
Ankle	6.3 ms	2.6 mV	Abductor hallucis-Ankle	6.3 ms	80 mm	m/s
Knee	15.8 ms	1.0 mV	Ankle-Knee	9.5 ms	360 mm	38 m/s
Median L						
Wrist	12.1 ms	5.0 mV	Abductor pollicis brevis-Wrist	12.1 ms	70 mm	m/s
Elbow	17.2 ms	5.1 mV	Wrist-Elbow	5.1 ms	220 mm	43 m/s
Ulnar L						
Wrist	3.3 ms	9.9 mV	Abductor digiti minimi (manus)-Wrist	3.3 ms	60 mm	18 m/s
Below elbow	7.4 ms	7.9 mV	Wrist-Below elbow	4.1 ms	230 mm	56 m/s
Above elbow	9.7 ms	7.7 mV	Below elbow-Above elbow	2.3 ms	90 mm	39 m/s
Median R						
Wrist	14.6 ms	3.2 mV	Abductor pollicis brevis-Wrist	14.6 ms	70 mm	m/s
Elbow	19.6 ms	2.5 mV	Wrist-Elbow	5.0 ms	228 mm	46 m/s
Ulnar R						
Wrist	3.9 ms	9.2 mV	Abductor digiti minimi (manus)-Wrist	3.9 ms	60 mm	15 m/s
Below elbow	8.1 ms	8.6 mV	Wrist-Below elbow	4.2 ms	223 mm	53 m/s
Above elbow	10.0 ms	9.8 mV	Below elbow-Above elbow	1.9 ms	73 mm	38 m/s

F-Wave Studies

Nerve	M-Latency	F-Latency
Tibial L	7.3	61.4

Sensory Nerve Conduction:

Nerve and Site	Onset Latency	Peak Latency	Amplitude	Segment	Latency Difference	Distance	Conduction Velocity
Sural L							
Lower leg (sural)	2.7 ms	3.3 ms	7 mV	Ankle (sural) - lower leg (sural)	2.7 ms	100 mm	37 m/s
Superficial peroneal L							
Lower leg (superficial peroneal)	2.8 ms	3.7 ms	5 mV	Ankle (superficial peroneal) - low leg (superficial peroneal)	2.8 ms	115 mm	41 m/s
Sural R							
Lower leg (sural)	2.9 ms	3.3 ms	6 mV	Ankle (sural) - lower leg (sural)	2.9 ms	100 mm	35 m/s
Superficial peroneal R							
Lower leg (superficial peroneal)	2.5 ms	3.1 ms	4 mV	Ankle (superficial peroneal) - low leg (superficial peroneal)	2.5 ms	110 mm	44 m/s
Median R							
Digit II	4.8 ms	5.3 ms	1 mV	Wrist – digit II	4.8 ms	125 mm	26 m/s
Ulnar R							
Digit V	2.7 ms	3.3 ms	3 mV	Wrist – digit V	2.7 ms	107 mm	40 m/s
Median L							
Digit II	No response						
Ulnar L							
Digit V	2.4 ms	2.9 ms	4 mV	Wrist – digit V	2.4 ms	103 mm	43 m/s

FIGURE 19-1 Nerve conduction studies from the patient with recurrent mononeuropathies.

If a sural nerve biopsy is performed it may demonstrate evidence of demyelination and "tomaculous" change (focal, sausage-like enlargement of the nerve), although this finding is not specific for HNPP.

In 80% of individuals affected by HNPP there will be a 1.5-Mb deletion at 17p11.2 that includes the *PMP22* gene. In contrast, a 1.5-Mb duplication is responsible for Charcot-Marie-Tooth neuropathy type 1A (see chapter 18, this volume). Therefore, HNPP is likely to be the consequence of a gene dosage effect (e.g. a deficiency of peripheral myelin protein 22 or PMP22; van de Wetering et al., 2002). Additionally, approximately 20% of families with HNPP will have a variety of *PMP22* point mutations that produce frame shifts, premature termination of translation, or other abnormalities.

After genetic counseling, the patient decides to have genetic testing, revealing the 1.5-Mb deletion at 17p11.2 that encompassing the *PMP22* gene. He was given a wrist splint for his symptoms of carpal tunnel syndrome. He was also advised to use protective pads at the elbows and knees to prevent pressure and trauma to local nerves. It was recommended that he avoid prolonged sitting with his legs crossed, prolonged leaning on his elbows, repetitive movements of the wrist, rapid weight loss, and medications that are potentially toxic to peripheral nerves (e.g. vincristine). He was not referred for surgical management, since spontaneous recovery is common and there is no evidence of a beneficial outcome from surgery. Genetic counselling and genetic testing was also provided to other affected family members, which showed the same genetic abnormality.

KEY POINTS TO REMEMBER ABOUT HEREDITARY NEUROPATHY WITH LIABILITY TO PRESSURE PALSIES

- The diagnosis of hereditary neuropathy with liability to pressure palsies (HNPP) should be considered when patients have recurrent focal compressive neuropathies with a family history consistent with autosomal dominant inheritance.
- Other clinical findings include the absence of ankle reflexes, a diffuse reduction in deep tendon reflexes, and a mild to moderate pes cavus foot deformity.

- Key findings on electrodiagnostic studies include bilateral slowing of sensory and motor median nerve conduction at the carpal tunnel with at least one abnormal parameter for motor conduction in one peroneal nerve.
- The underlying molecular defect, which is present in 80% of affected individuals, is a 1.5-Mb deletion at 17p11.2 that includes the *PMP22* gene.
- Treatments include wrist splints for carpal tunnel syndrome and avoidance of activities that put pressure and trauma on local nerves.

Further Reading

Bird TD. Hereditary Neuropathy with Liability to Pressure Palsies. In: Pagon RA, Adam MP, Bird TD, Dolan CR, Fong CT, Stephens K, eds. GeneReviews. Seattle, WA.

Mouton, P., Tardieu, S., Gouider, R., Birouk, N., Maisonobe, T., Dubourg, O.,... & Bouche, P. (1999). Spectrum of clinical and electrophysiologic features in HNPP patients with the 17p11.2 deletion. *Neurology*, *52*, 1440–1446.

van de Wetering, R. A., Gabreels-Festen, A. A., Timmerman, V., Padberg, G. M., Gabreels, F. J., & Mariman, E. C. (2002). Hereditary neuropathy with liability to pressure palsies with a small deletion interrupting the *PMP22* gene. *Neuromuscular Disorders: NMD*, *12*, 651–655.

20 Neurofibromatosis Type 1

A 52-year-old lady was referred to your neurogenetics clinic for assessment of neurofibromatosis.

She has a history of extensive cutaneous neurofibromas from early adulthood. She has had six neurofibroma resections for larger or painful lesions.

The patient is the third of four siblings. Her older sister and father are also affected by neurofibromatosis. Her sister had a tumor resected at the C2 vertebrae and has been troubled by scoliosis. No other family members are known to be affected and the patient does not have any children.

On examination, there were extensive cutaneous neurofibromas covering the skin surface (Figure 20-1.)

There were at least four or five café au lait spots over the torso and legs. She had no signs of plexiform neurofibromas or scoliosis.

What do you do now?

The patient has many of the characteristic clinical features of neurofibromatosis 1 (NF1) or von Recklinghausen disease. The clinical diagnosis of NF1 is based on at least two major features out of the following seven: (1) a first degree relative with NF1, (2) six or more café au lait patches that may either be present at birth or otherwise appear in the first few years of life, (3) axillary or groin freckling, (4) Lisch nodules in the iris, (5) optic pathway glioma, (6) bony dysplasia of the sphenoid wing, and (7) pseudarthrosis of the long bones (Ferner, 2010).

Neurofibromas are benign peripheral nerve-sheath tumors. They can manifest as localized cutaneous and subcutaneous growths, spinal nerve root tumors and plexiform lesions. Cutaneous neurofibromas develop in the majority of patients, usually in early adulthood, but can appear in childhood. Cutaneous lesions can lead to considerable psychological distress. However, unlike subcutaneous and plexiform neurofibromas, they do not undergo malignant change. Subcutaneous neurofibromas are peripheral nerve tumors that often cause pain and neurological deficit. Women who develop subcutaneous breast lumps should be referred to a specialized breast unit given that it may be difficult to distinguish carcinoma from neurofibroma, and NF1 females have increased susceptibility for developing breast cancer before the age of 50 years. About 60% of patients affected by NF1 develop plexiform neurofibromas that can cause neurological deficit and

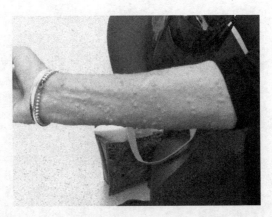

FIGURE 20-1 Photograph of the patient's right arm demonstrating extensive cutaneous neurofibromas.

disfigurement. Plexiform neurofibromas are difficult to manage since surgical treatment is often unsatisfactory (Friedman, 1993).

Malignant peripheral nerve-sheath tumors typically arise from preexisting focal subcutaneous neurofibromas or plexiform neurofibromas, but they can also develop de novo. Malignant peripheral nerve-sheath tumors can be challenging to diagnose given that they occur in individuals who are accustomed to developing lumps, and they can be difficult to distinguish from benign tumors. They should be suspected if any of the following symptoms arise: (a) persistent or nocturnal pain associated with a plexiform or subcutaneous neurofibroma, (b) a rapid increase in size of a neurofibroma, (c) a new or unexplained neurological deficit, and (c) a change in texture (e.g., increasing hardness) of a neurofibroma.

Spinal nerve root neurofibromas can be asymptomatic or cause pressure on the adjacent spinal nerve root or spinal cord. Patients with NF1 can also suffer from numerous other manifestations such as an axonal symmetrical neurofibromatous neuropathy, cerebral malformations (e.g., Chiari 1 malformation and aqueduct stenosis), epilepsy, cognitive impairment, multiple sclerosis, brain and optic pathway tumors, asymptomatic iris Lisch nodules, bony abnormalities (e.g., short stature, pseudarthrosis of the long bones, scoliosis), cardiovascular disease (part of the NF1 vasculopathy spectrum), respiratory complications, gastrointestinal complications, and pheochromocytoma.

The diagnosis of NF1 is usually based on clinical findings, and molecular genetic testing is rarely required. However, prenatal diagnosis or preimplantation genetic diagnosis may be needed for at-risk pregnancies, and this requires prior identification of the disease-causing mutation in the family. NF1 is an autosomal dominant disorder in which heterozygous mutations of the *NF1* gene are responsible for the vast majority of cases. Half of affected individuals have NF1 as a consequence of a de novo mutation in the *NF1* gene. Sequencing analysis will detect about 90% of *NF1* intragenic mutations. A further 4–5% of patients will have whole gene deletions, which can be identified using different methods including multiple ligation-dependent probe amplification (MLPA).

The diagnosis of NF1 can be confused with another dominantly inherited disorder known as Legius syndrome. This is a condition that includes multiple café-au-lait spots, axillary freckling, macrocephaly and sometimes

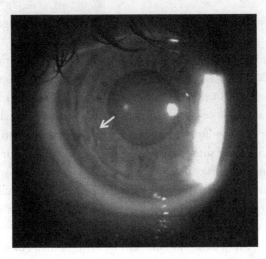

FIGURE 20-2 Photograph of the patient's eye demonstrating Lisch nodules in the iris (arrow).

facial features that resemble Noonan syndrome. It is caused by heterozygous mutations in the *SPRED1* gene. Affected individuals may meet the diagnostic criteria for NF1, but certain clinical features such as Lisch nodules, neurofibromas, and central nervous system tumors do not usually occur.

The patient was referred for an ophthalmology review for slit lamp assessment (Figure 20-2).

Although the patient was not planning on starting a family, the decision was made to proceed with genetic testing. The *NF1* and *SPRED1* genes were analyzed by polymerase chain reaction and sequencing of both strands of the entire coding region and exon-intron splice junctions. In addition, MLPA was performed to test for deletions or duplications of the *NF1* and *SPRED1* genes.

Sequencing of the *NF1* gene revealed a previously unreported heterozygous change in exon 51 of the *NF1* gene (c.7586delC, p.Pro2529Leufs*19). The c.7586delC deletion creates a shift in the reading frame starting at codon 2529. The new reading frame ends in a stop codon 18 positions downstream, which is very likely to result in a truncated protein or loss of protein production. No mutations were detected in the *SPRED1* gene.

You advise the patient that she will need to be seen on a regular basis (at least annually) in your clinic for monitoring of complications. You note that the patient has recently had magnetic resonance imaging (MRI) of the brain which did not show any evidence of an optic pathway glioma or any other structural lesions. You also warn the patient to contact you if she develops any suspicious symptoms (such as symptoms suggestive of malignant peripheral nerve sheath tumors, or if she notices a breast lump, etc.).

KEY POINTS TO REMEMBER ABOUT NEUROFIBROMATOSIS TYPE 1

- The clinical diagnosis of neurofibromatosis type 1 (NF1) is based on at least two major features out of the following seven: (1) a first degree relative with NF1, (2) six or more café au lait patches, which may either be present at birth or otherwise appear in the first few years of life, (3) axillary or groin freckling, (4) Lisch nodules in the iris, (5) optic pathway glioma, (6) bony dysplasia of the sphenoid wing, (7) pseudarthrosis of the long bones.
- The neurofibromas can manifest as localized cutaneous and subcutaneous growths, spinal nerve root tumors, and plexiform lesions.
- Malignant peripheral nerve-sheath tumors should be suspected if one of the following symptoms arise: (a) persistent or nocturnal pain associated with a plexiform or subcutaneous neurofibroma, (b) a rapid increase in size of a neurofibroma, (c) a new or unexplained neurological deficit, and (d) the neurofibroma changes to a hard texture.
- The majority of cases are cause by mutations in the *NF1* gene although molecular genetic testing is usually not required to confirm the diagnosis.

Further Reading

Ferner, R. E. (2010). The neurofibromatoses. *Practical Neurology, 10,* 82–93.

Friedman, J. M. (1993). Neurofibromatosis 1. In R. A. Pagon, M. P. Adam, T. D. Bird, C. R. Dolan, C. T. Fong, & K. Stephens (Eds.), *GeneReviews.* Seattle, WA: University of Washington.

21 The Myotonic Dystrophies

This 58-year-old man presented to the neurogenetics clinic for evaluation of myotonic dystrophy. He noticed that his muscles had been "feeling tired" since his fifth decade. He now has difficulty walking and trouble climbing stairs and standing for prolonged periods of time. He has had multiple falls, often when using the stairs.

His past medical history includes hypertension, hypercholesterolemia, and type 2 diabetes mellitus complicated by diabetic nephropathy. Additionally, he has a history of cataracts requiring cataract surgery several years ago.

The only family history of note is that his father had a history of premature baldness, and toward the end of his life he was unable to sign his name due to tremulousness of his hands.

On examination, the patient had frontal balding with atrophy of the temporalis and masseter muscles. There was mild ptosis bilaterally. There was evidence of facial weakness as well as mild weakness of neck flexion. Examination of the upper and lower limbs revealed predominantly proximal weakness, most pronounced for shoulder abduction and hip flexion. Deep tendon reflexes were present except for the right ankle jerk and sensory modalities were normal. There was some contraction myotonia seen but percussion myotonia could not be elicited.

He previously had a needle electromyography (EMG), which showed evidence of myotonia. He does not think he has ever had genetic testing but is interested in pursuing this option.

What do you do now?

The patient appears to have a clinical phenotype consistent with myotonic dystrophy. The myotonic dystrophies are characterised by progressive muscle degeneration leading to disabling weakness and wasting with myotonia (i.e., delayed relaxation or prolonged contraction of skeletal muscle), in combination with multisystem involvement.

There are two major types of myotonic dystrophy: type 1 (also known as Steinert disease), and type 2 (also known as proximal myotonic myopathy or PROMM). Both diseases are caused by autosomal dominant nucleotide repeat expansions. In patients with myotonic dystrophy type 1, a $(CTG)_n$ expansion is present in *DMPK* gene, whereas, in patients with type 2 disease, there is a $(CCTG)_n$ expansion in *CNBP/ZNF9* gene (Ude & Krahe, 2012). It can be difficult to distinguish between adult onset type 1 myotonic dystrophy and type 2 myotonic dystrophy, but there are some features from the clinical vignette that favor type 2 disease.

The clinical phenotype in myotonic dystrophy type 2 is highly variable, ranging from progressive disability from the age of 40 years, early cardiac death, or mild proximal weakness to a slight elevation in the creatine kinase concentration in elderly patients. The first subjective symptom of muscle disease is usually either proximal lower limb weakness, causing difficulties with climbing stairs, or myalgic pains. Typical features of myotonic dystrophy type 1, such as myotonia, can be absent in patients with type 2 disease. Compared to type 1 disease, type 2 disease has a later age of symptom onset, the clinical course is more favorable, and the life expectancy is close to normal. Furthermore, in type 2 disease, there is usually no prominent respiratory, facial, or bulbar weakness. However, severe variants of type 2 disease sometimes do occur, with manifestations including fatal cardiac arrhythmias, respiratory failure, progressive muscular atrophy, and marked disability.

In this case, the pattern of weakness was predominantly proximal and, therefore, favors a diagnosis of myotonic dystrophy type 2. It is unclear whether his father was affected; for example, his father was prematurely bald and frontal baldness can be a rare manifestation of type 2 disease.

Genetic testing in the patient described in the clinical vignette detected the presence of an expanded allele on intron 1 of the *CNBP* gene, confirming the diagnosis of myotonic dystrophy type 2. In order to investigate for cardiac arrhythmias, the patient had an electrocardiogram and cardiac

Holter monitor, which revealed atrial and ventricular ectopics only. The patient was referred to physiotherapy, occupational therapy, and social services.

The patient also received genetic counseling. It is notable that each child of an individual with a *CNBP* expansion has a 50% chance of inheriting the expansion (Dalton, Ranum, & Day, 1993). Disease severity, age at onset, and clinical symptoms cannot be predicted according to the size of the expanded allele. Prenatal testing can be considered if the presence of a *CNBP* expansion has been identified in the affected parent.

KEY POINTS TO REMEMBER ABOUT THE MYOTONIC DYSTROPHIES

- The myotonic dystrophies are characterized by progressive muscle degeneration leading to disabling weakness and wasting with myotonia, in combination with multisystem involvement.
- There are two major types of myotonic dystrophy: type 1 and type 2.
- In patients with myotonic dystrophy type 1, a $(CTG)_n$ expansion is present in *DMPK* gene, whereas in patients with type 2 disease, there is a $(CCTG)_n$ expansion in *CNBP/ZNF9* gene.
- Compared to type 1 disease, type 2 disease has a proximal rather than distal pattern of weakness, respiratory or bulbar weakness occurs less frequently, there is a later age of symptom onset, the clinical course is more favorable, and the life expectancy is close to normal.

Further Reading

Ude, B., & Krahe, R. (2012). The myotonic dystrophies: molecular, clinical, and therapeutic challenges. *Lancet Neurology*, *11*, 891–905.

Dalton, J. C., Ranum, L. P. W/, Day, J. W. (1993). Myotonic dystrophy type 2. In R. A. Pagon, M. P. Adam, T. D. Bird, C. R. Dolan, C. T. Fong, & K. Stephens (Eds.) *GeneReviews*. Seattle, WA: University of Washington.

22 The Dystrophinopathies

A 32-year-old man with Becker muscular dystrophy is referred to the neurogenetics clinic.

The patient is one of two sons of unrelated parents. There is no family history of Becker muscular dystrophy. He was found to have a missense mutation in exon 69 of the *DMD* gene (involving c.10003 in codon 3335). The patient's mother was identified as a carrier of this disorder.

The patient had a normal birth and early childhood development. He first noticed muscle weakness from the age of 11 years. This slowly progressed over time and now has affected his gait, with particular difficulty walking up an incline. He is unable to rise from a chair without assistance, and has difficulty getting in and out of cars. He also feels that his arms get tired easily. There are no bulbar, respiratory, or cardiac symptoms.

Important findings on examination include marked scapular winging, proximal upper limb weakness, and diffuse weakness and areflexia of the lower limbs. Gait examination reveals a waddling gait with bilateral foot drop.

He is interested in genetic counseling (he wishes to start a family) and the ongoing management of his muscular dystrophy.

What do you do now?

The dystrophinopathies include a spectrum of muscle disorders and are inherited in an X-linked fashion. They are caused by mutations in the *DMD* gene, which is located on the X chromosome and encodes for the dystrophin protein. At the mild end of the disease severity, patients may have an asymptomatic increase in serum creatine kinase, muscle cramps, and myoglobinuria, or isolated myopathy of the quadriceps muscle. At the severe end of the disease spectrum there are progressive muscle diseases called Duchenne or Becker muscular dystrophy when skeletal muscle is primarily involved and *DMD*-associated dilated cardiomyopathy when the heart is primarily affected (Darras, Miller, & Urion, 1993).

Duchenne muscular dystrophy usually presents in early childhood with delayed milestones, such as delays in sitting and standing independently. Patients may have a waddling gait and difficulty climbing up stairs due to proximal muscle weakness. This condition may progress rapidly, leaving affected children wheelchair dependent by the age of 12 years. Duchenne muscular dystrophy is usually complicated by cardiomyopathy after 18 years of age. Few patients will survive beyond the third decade, with respiratory complications and cardiomyopathy being the most common cause of death.

Compared to Duchenne muscular dystrophy, Becker muscular dystrophy has a milder phenotype with later-onset of the skeletal muscle weakness. Individuals with this condition can remain ambulatory into their 20s. Although the skeletal muscle weakness is milder, heart failure is a common cause of morbidity and mortality, with the mean age of death being in the mid-40s. The *DMD*-associated cardiomyopathy is characterized by left ventricular dilatation and congestive cardiac failure. Female carriers are also at increased risk of cardiomyopathy.

The diagnosis of dystrophinopathies can nearly always be made by molecular genetic testing of the *DMD* gene, although in some cases a combination of clinical findings, family history, serum creatine kinase and muscle biopsy with dystrophin studies are required to confirm the diagnosis.

You explain the concept of an X-linked inherited disorder to the patient. You tell him that all his sons will inherit his Y chromosome, and so none of his boys will be affected by Becker muscular dystrophy. In contrast, all of his daughters will inherit his X chromosome, and so will be obligate carriers of the mutation. Although it is very unlikely that any of his girls will manifest with symptoms of the Becker muscular dystrophy, they are still at risk of cardiomyopathy and so will require cardiac surveillance later in life. His daughters will have a 50% chance of passing on the disease-causing mutation with each of their pregnancies, and they may be candidates for prenatal genetic testing.

A critical part of his management is surveillance transthoracic echo-cardiograms for cardiomyopathy. Once developed, cardiomyopathy and congestive heart failure in the Duchenne and Becker muscular dystrophy populations are managed with medical and device management similar to other forms of cardiomyopathy. For patients with Becker muscular dystrophy, cardiac transplant may be considered (Romfh & McNally, 2010).

The patient from the clinical vignette was found to have right bundle branch block on electrocardiogram, but no serious cardiac arrhythmias were found on Holter monitoring. Transthoracic echocardiogram showed some septal dyssynergic motion but normal biventricular size and overall systolic function. Additionally, pulmonary function tests were performed and did not show any major abnormalities.

The skeletal muscle may be more susceptible to contraction-induced muscle-fiber injury in patients with dystrophinopathies, and so it may be better to avoid certain types of strenuous exercise (Bushby et al., 2010). With this in mind you strongly recommend low impact exercises such as swimming and cycling. You also suggest that he should stop exercising if he feels tired or if his muscles get sore.

Evidence from randomized controlled studies have shown that cortico-steroid therapy in Duchenne muscular dystrophy improves muscle strength and function in the short-term (Manzur, Kuntzer, Pike, & Swan, 2004). The most effective prednisolone regime appears to be 0.75 mg/kg/day. After discussing this with the patient, you start him on a trial of prednisolone using a dosage appropriate for his weight.

KEY POINTS TO REMEMBER ABOUT THE DYSTROPHINOPATHIES

- The dystrophinopathies include a spectrum of muscle disorders causes by mutations in the *DMD* gene, which encodes for the dystrophin protein.
- They have an X-linked mode of inheritance.

- Involvement of skeletal muscle can cause progressive muscle disease (Duchenne or Becker muscular dystrophy).
- Involvement of the heart can cause *DMD*-associated dilated cardiomyopathy.
- Management includes surveillance and prompt treatment of cardiopulmonary complications, and patients may also benefit from the administration of corticosteroids.

Further Reading

Bushby, K., Finkel, R., Birnkrant, D. J., Case, L. E., Clemens, P. R., Cripe, L.,... & Constantin, C. (2010). Diagnosis and management of Duchenne muscular dystrophy, part 2: Implementation of multidisciplinary care. *Lancet Neurology*, 9, 177–189.

Darras, B. T., Miller, D. T., & Urion, D. K. (1993). Dystrophinopathies. In R. A. Pagon, M. P. Adam, T. D. Bird, C. R. Dolan, C. T. Fong, & K. Stephens (Eds), *GeneReviews*. Seattle, WA: University of Washington.

Manzur, A. Y., Kuntzer, T., Pike, M., & Swan, A. (2004). Glucocorticoid corticosteroids for Duchenne muscular dystrophy. *Cochrane Database of Systematic Reviews*, 2, CD003725.

Romfh, A., & McNally, E. M. (2010). Cardiac assessment in duchenne and becker muscular dystrophies. *Current Heart Failure Reports*, 7, 212–218.

23 Facioscapulohumeral Dystrophy

A 50-year-old woman was referred with a long-standing history of weakness in the legs with difficulty running and playing sports. She also found it hard to walk up and down stairs. Additionally, she had trouble lifting her arms above her head. She noticed that she could no longer smile and also had symptoms of dyspnea and dysphagia. She recently noticed hearing loss in the right ear following a flight to a nearby city.

The family history was remarkable for the fact that the patient's two daughters had similar symptoms.

On examination, there was evidence of bilateral facial weakness with absence of wrinkling of the forehead, weakness of eye closure, and a horizontal smile with inability to purse the lips or whistle. The extraocular eye movements were intact and her speech was normal. There was evidence of bilateral scapular winging with weakness of elbow flexion and extension in both upper limbs. There was also weakness of ankle dorsiflexion in the lower limbs. The deep tendon reflexes were normal throughout and sensation was intact. Beevor sign was negative. She has difficulty rising from the squatting position or from low chairs.

What do you do now?

The clinical vignette demonstrates some typical features of facioscapulo-humeral dystrophy (FSHD). This is an autosomal dominant disorder with symptom onset occurring most often in the second decade of life, although disease onset can range from infancy to late adulthood.

As the name implies, there is a specific anatomical distribution to the weakness in FSHD, a feature that aids in the clinical diagnosis. Initially, weakness is often limited to the face (Farmakidis, 2011). Facial weakness can involve weakness of eye closure, a horizontal smile, and inability to purse the lips or whistle. Facial weakness is usually followed by weakness of the muscles around the scapulae, resulting in difficulty raising the arms and scapular winging. The humeral component of FSHD refers to weakness of the biceps and triceps. A typical pattern of wasting of certain muscles and relatively preserved bulk in other muscles, along with bony prominences, leads to the so called "poly-hill" sign in FSHD (Pradhan, 2002).

Although weakness is characteristically proximal in the upper limbs, weakness in the lower extremities usually begins distally in muscles such as the tibialis anterior and may result in a foot drop (Farmakidis, 2011). Beevor sign is common in patients with a classical FSHD phenotype and involves upward deflection of the umbilicus on flexion of the neck (Eger, Jordan, Habermann, & Zierz, 2010). It is due to paralysis of the inferior portion of the rectus abdominis muscle, so that the upper muscle fibers predominate, pulling the umbilicus upward.

Extramuscular manifestations can also occur in FSHD and include high-frequency hearing loss and retinal vascular malformations. The retinal vascular abnormalities may progress to exudative retinopathy and visual impairment, a condition known as Coats disease.

The patient described in the clinical vignette has a pattern of weakness that could be consistent with FSHD. There is also a positive family history in keeping with autosomal dominant transmission, and a known extramuscular manifestation of FSHD (i.e., hearing loss). However, it is somewhat unusual that the patient has prominent dysphagia and respiratory symptoms given that bulbar, respiratory, and cardiac involvement is rare in this condition (Farmakidis, 2011).

Routine laboratory investigations are important in this circumstance and include measurement of the creatine kinase (CK) levels. The CK can be mildly elevated in FSHD, but if it is greater than 10 times normal, an alternative condition should be suspected (Farmakidis, 2011). Nerve conduction studies and electromyography may also be useful (e.g., can help distinguish between neurogenic and myopathic causes of scapular winging). Muscle biopsy typically shows nonspecific findings in FSHD and may not be required if genetic testing is available.

The large majority (more than 95%) of patients with FSHD have a partial deletion of one of their chromosome 4 repeat arrays (D4Z4; Tawil, van der Maarel, Padberg, & van Engelen, 2010). This repeat array is polymorphic in copy number, with alleles varying between 11 and 100 units in the general population. Patients with FSHD1 will carry one allele with 1-10 D4Z4 units. In order to be pathogenic, this repeat array needs to be located on the 4qA background of chromosome 4 rather than the similar repeat array on chromosome 10 and chromosome 4qB. Genetic confirmation of FSHD1 is routinely done on peripheral blood lymphocyte DNA by Southern blotting and hybridization of a set of probes to allow for the establishment of the size of the repeat array on 4q35 and to determine the genetic background of chromosome 4q (e.g. A or B; Tawil et al., 2010). In unaffected individuals, this method will show two 4q35 alleles of >50 Kb on the basis of digestion with *Eco*RI/*Bln*I restriction enzymes, whereas in affected individuals the 4q35 allele will be between 10 and 38 Kb, with intermediate values considered inconclusive. This test is highly sensitive and specific; however, false positives will affect a minority (<5%) of patients.

In the presenting patient, genetic testing for FSHD revealed that one allele exhibited a 16 Kb fragment length, which is well within the affected range, confirming the diagnosis.

Respiratory failure can occur in FSHD but is rare, affecting only about 1% of patients (Wohlgemuth, van der Koi, vanKesteren, van der Maarel, & Padberg, 2004). However, clinicians need to be aware of this complication, since unrecognized and untreated respiratory failure can unexpectedly lead to early mortality (Tawil, 2010).

Given the patient's symptoms of shortness of breath, pulmonary function testing was performed. The patient's lung function tests revealed evidence of a restrictive ventilatory defect and the patient was referred to a respiratory physician for further management.

Although there are no disease-specific therapies available for FSHD, it is important to treat the symptoms and screen for complications. It is recommended that all patients with FSHD who are experiencing limitations be referred for an initial rehabilitation consult (Tawil et al., 2010). Aerobic training may also be beneficial in patients with FSHD (Olsen, Orngreen, & Vissing, 2005). FSHD is frequently complicated by pain, and this should be treated appropriately. Screening for respiratory dysfunction is recommended in patients with moderate to severe disease. Some patients at high risk of respiratory impairment (e.g., those who are wheelchair-dependent, those who have pelvic girdle weakness, superimposed pulmonary disease, moderate to severe kyphoscoliosis, lumber hyperlordosis, or chest wall abnormalities) should have yearly forced vital-capacity measurements (Tawil, 2010). Individuals with ventilatory defects may require noninvasive ventilatory support.

Patients may also need testing and treatment for hearing loss, since this may lead to delayed language development if this complication is overlooked in infantile-onset disease. All patients with FSHD should also be referred to an ophthalmologist since retinal vasculopathy is treatable using laser therapy of pathologically dilated retinal vessels (Tawil, 2010).

Prenatal diagnosis is possible in FSHD, but many patients do not request this option given that the condition is usually mild. Pre-implantation genetic diagnosis is also potentially available but is difficult because the testing is not polymerase chain-reaction-based and, therefore, requires more DNA than can be obtained from a single cell. Pre-implantation genetic diagnosis can also be inferred using linkage analysis of multiple family members, but the effectiveness of this approach is not clear.

KEY POINTS TO REMEMBER ABOUT FACIOSCAPULOHUMERAL DYSTROPHY

- There is a selective pattern of weakness in facioscapulohumeral dystrophy (FSHD) with involvement of face, shoulder (producing scapular winging), biceps, triceps and tibialis anterior.
- Respiratory involvement is rare but can lead to early and unexpected mortality if unrecognized—patients at high risk should undergo lung function screening tests.
- Extramuscular complications of FSHD include hearing impairment and retinal vasculopathy.
- The large majority (more than 95%) of patients with FSHD have a partial deletion of one of their chromosome 4 repeat arrays (D4Z4).

Further Reading

Pradhan, S. (2002). Poly-Hill sign in facioscapulohumeral dystrophy. *Muscle & Nerve, 25,* 754–755.

Eger, K., Jordan, B., Habermann, S., & Zierz, S. (2010). Beevor's sign in facioscapulohumeral muscular dystrophy: An old sign with new implications. *Journal of Neurology, 257,* 436–438.

Farmakidis, C. T. R. (2011). Facioscapulohumeral dystrophy. In R. N. V. S. Tawil (Ed.), Neuromuscular disorders (pp. 75–79). Hoboken, NJ: John Wiley & Sons.

Olsen, D. B., Orngreen, M. C., & Vissing, J. (2005). Aerobic training improves exercise performance in facioscapulohumeral muscular dystrophy. *Neurology, 64,* 1064–1066.

Tawil, R., van der Maarel, S., Padberg, G. W., & van Engelen, B. G. (2010). 171st ENMC international workshop: Standards of care and management of facioscapulohumeral muscular dystrophy. *Neuromuscular Disorders: NMD, 20,* 471–475.

Wohlgemuth, M., van der Kooi, E. L., van Kesteren, R. G., van der Maarel, S. M., & Padberg, G. W. (2004).Ventilatory support in facioscapulohumeral muscular dystrophy. *Neurology, 63,* 176–178.

24 Inclusion Body Myopathy with Paget Disease of Bone and/or Frontotemporal Dementia

A 44-year-old man presents to your clinic with a four-year history of aching pain "all over the body," but particularly in the hips and lower back (previously reported by Kumar et al., 2010). He also complains of difficulty getting out of chairs and climbing up and down stairs.

On examination of the upper limbs, you notice fasciculations in the triceps bilaterally. He has scapular winging and weakness of shoulder abduction and external rotation. There is also spasticity with hyperreflexia. On examination of the lower limbs, there was bilateral wasting of the calves and weakness of hip flexion. There was moderate spasticity bilaterally and the knee reflexes and left ankle reflex were exaggerated. The right ankle reflex was reduced and the plantar responses were flexor. On gait examination, the patient had a waddling gait as well as camptocormia and a positive Trendelenburg sign bilaterally. He did not have any cranial nerve, cerebellar, or sensory signs, and cognitive testing with the Mini-Mental State Examination and Frontal Assessment Battery was normal.

The patient's 35-year-old brother was present during the appointment and was experiencing similar symptoms. He noticed increasing difficulty carrying heavy items up and down stairs, weakness of his legs, and difficulty running. Salient examination findings included bilateral scapular winging, wasting of the biceps and clavicular head of pectoralis, weakness of shoulder abduction and external rotation, wasting of the left calf, hip flexion weakness, absent ankle jerks, and a waddling gait.

On further question, you are interested to find that the proband's mother also suffered from neurological symptoms, including difficulty climbing stairs and getting out of chairs. Review of the medical records documented a physical examination performed in her mid-40s reporting signs of bilateral winging of the scapula, difficulty rising from squatting and proximal limb weakness. Deep tendon reflexes were described as "brisk." She was given a diagnosis of amyotrophic lateral sclerosis (ALS). She was also diagnosed with severe Paget disease of the bone, which particularly affected her legs, shoulders, and neck. Furthermore, she developed progressive cognitive impairment in her late 40s. By 53 years of age, she was profoundly demented with severe behavioral and communication difficulties. She died at the age of 55 years from respiratory complications; an autopsy was not performed.

What do you do now?

The clinical phenotype in this family is complex. The proband appears to have a myopathic process with a predominantly proximal pattern of weakness. However, there are also corticospinal tract signs, and together with the presence of fasciculations, raise the possibility of anterior horn cell disease (e.g. ALS). It is likely that his brother and mother are affected by the same condition, with a mode of inheritance that could be autosomal dominant or even mitochondrial (maternal). You pay particular attention to the history of Paget disease and early-onset dementia in the patient's mother, and recognize that the clinical phenotype in this family could be explained by a condition called *inclusion body myopathy* with *Paget* disease of bone and/or *frontotemporal dementia* (IBMPFD).

IBMPFD is a progressive, fatal disorder with variable penetrance chiefly affecting three main tissue types: muscle (IBM), bone (Paget disease of bone), and brain (frontotemporal dementia; Nalbandian, et al., 2011). It has an autosomal dominant mode of inheritance and is caused by mutations in the *valosin-containing protein* (*VCP*) gene. Most individuals who develop IBM suffer from progressive proximal muscle weakness. Muscle biopsies typically reveal rimmed vacuoles and inclusions that are ubiquitin- and TAR DNA binding protein-43 (TDP-43)-positive on immunohistochemistry. Paget disease of bone, which is seen in about half of the cases, is caused by overactive osteoclasts and is associated clinically with pain, an elevated serum alkaline phosphatase (ALP), and X-ray findings of coarse trabeculation and sclerotic lesions. Frontotemporal dementia is diagnosed at a mean age of 55 years in a third of individuals and is characterized clinically by deficits in comprehension, naming, calculation, and social awareness. Additionally, it is now apparent that the clinical spectrum of IBMPFD includes phenotypes that closely resemble motor neurone disease, and that *VCP* mutations account for approximately 1–2% of cases of familial ALS (Johnson et al., 2010).

You order nerve conduction studies for the proband and the patient's brother, which reveal normal motor, sensory and long-latency responses. Findings on needle electromyography include occasional fasciculations, with signs of chronic denervation and partial reinnervation in the muscles of the shoulder girdle and limbs, without any myopathic features.

You order a muscle biopsy in the patient's brother (Figure 24-1).

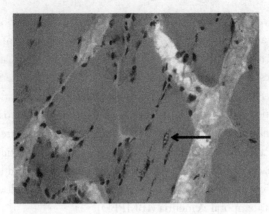

FIGURE 24-1 Muscle biopsy with hematoxylin and eosin staining from the proband's brother. A rimmed vacuole is indicated by the black arrow. Adapted from a figure by Kumar et al. (2010) (with permission from Science Direct).

The muscle biopsy appears to confirm changes consistent with inclusion body myositis. Electron microscopy showed evidence of inclusion body myositis type filaments associated with some of the rimmed vacuoles. Immunostaining with TDP-43 revealed the presence of focal granular and filamentous cytoplasmic staining in a number of myofibers in a section of deltoid muscle.

You review the laboratory results, which included a mildly elevated creatine kinase in the proband (491 U/L, normal 10–140) as well as an elevated serum ALP level. You also order a whole body bone (WBBS) scan to investigate for Paget disease of bone (Figure 24-2).

The WBBS appears to show changes of Paget disease, which makes the diagnosis of IBMPFD highly likely. You request genetic testing of the *VCP* gene, which detects a novel mutation (c.464G>T, p.Arg155Leu). This mutation is likely to be pathogenic, because three other mutations at this site (Arg155His/Pro/Cys) account for a significant proportion of reported cases.

You provide the patient with genetic counseling and continue to see him in clinic. You monitor him for cognitive symptoms, since he is at high risk for developing frontotemporal dementia. He is given supportive management including treatment of Paget disease.

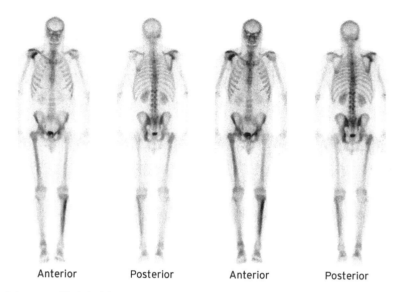

Anterior   Posterior   Anterior   Posterior

FIGURE 24-2 Whole body bone scan in the proband showing evidence of widespread Paget disease of bone with involvement of the right humerus, right femur, left tibia, and left hemipelvis. Adapted from a figure by Kumar et al. (2010) (with permission from Science Direct).

KEY POINTS TO REMEMBER ABOUT INCLUSION BODY MYOPATHY, WITH PAGET DISEASE OF BONE AND/OR FRONTOTEMPORAL DEMENTIA

- Inclusion body myopathy with Paget disease of bone and/or frontotemporal dementia (IBMPFD) is a progressive, fatal disorder with variable penetrance chiefly affecting three main tissue types: muscle (IBM), bone (Paget disease of bone), and brain (frontotemporal dementia).
- IBMPFD is an autosomal dominant condition caused by mutations in the *valosin-containing protein* (*VCP*) gene.
- IBMPFD should be included in the differential diagnosis for patients presenting with an amyotrophic lateral sclerosis-frontotemporal dementia syndrome.

Further Reading

Johnson, J. O., Mandrioli, J., Benatar, M., Abramzon, Y., Van Deerlin, V. M., Trojanowski, J. Q.,...& Traynor, B. J. (2010). Exome sequencing reveals VCP mutations as a cause of familial ALS. *Neuron, 68,* 857–864.

Kumar, K. R., Needham, M., Mina, K., Davis, M., Brewer, J., Staples, C.,...& Mastaglia, F. L. (2010). Two Australian families with inclusion-body myopathy, Paget's disease of bone and frontotemporal dementia: novel clinical and genetic findings. *Neuromuscular Disorders, 20,* 330–334.

Nalbandian, A., Donkervoort, S., Dec, E., Badadani, M., Katheria, V., Rana, P.,...& Kimonis, V. E. (2011). The multiple faces of valosin-containing protein-associated diseases: inclusion body myopathy with Paget's disease of bone, frontotemporal dementia, and amyotrophic lateral sclerosis. *Journal of Molecular Neuroscience, 45,* 522–531.

25 Hereditary Spastic Paraplegia

A 55-year-old man presents with a several year history of
unsteadiness of gait and stiffness in his legs. He also has
some symptoms of urinary urgency. He was found to have mild
cervical spinal stenosis on magnetic resonance imaging (MRI)
of his spine. He proceeded to a cervical spine decompression
but with no objective improvement in his symptoms or signs
postoperatively.

In terms of the family history, his brother and sister
are affected by a similar condition. There is no history of
consanguinity in the family.

On examination, he has saccadic intrusions into smooth
pursuit eye movements but no nystagmus. There was normal
tone, power, and reflexes in the upper limbs. Examination of the
lower limbs revealed moderate spasticity, with brisk reflexes
and extensor plantar responses but no weakness. There was
mild finger-nose and heel-shin ataxia. Sensation was normal
in the upper and lower limbs. His gait was unsteady due to a
combination of spasticity and ataxia.

He had a muscle biopsy that showed changes in keeping with
mitochondrial dysfunction (Figure 25-1).

He has received several diagnoses including multiple sclerosis;
however, his referring neurologist is still concerned about the
diagnosis and would like another opinion.

What do you do now?

The patient has signs of spasticity and ataxia. The differential diagnosis of a spastic-ataxia phenotype is broad and includes the spinocerebellar ataxias and hereditary spastic paraplegia (HSP) with ataxia. The findings on muscle biopsy (e.g., COX negative/SDH positive fibers) are suggestive of a mitochondrial etiology, pointing toward the spastic paraplegia 7 (SPG7) form of HSP as the most likely explanation for the presentation.

HSP can also be classified according to the clinical phenotype. In "pure" forms of HSP, the chief clinical feature is progressive spasticity in the lower limbs. Some additional neurological signs can be present such as sensory impairment in the legs and bladder symptoms. In "complicated" forms, major additional clinical features are present, such as cognitive impairment, seizures, dysarthria, cerebellar signs and peripheral neuropathy.

There is considerable genetic heterogeneity underlying HSP. In fact, at least 54 genes and 72 loci identified so far. Many of these HSP-causing genes have been discovered recently using whole exome sequencing (Novarino et al., 2014). The mode of inheritance in HSP can be autosomal dominant, autosomal recessive, X-linked or sporadic (Finsterer et al., 2012). The most common cause of autosomal dominant forms is SPG4, which is caused by mutations in the *SPAST* gene (Vendebona, Kerr, Liang, & Sue, 2012). Some autosomal recessive forms of HSP are frequently associated with

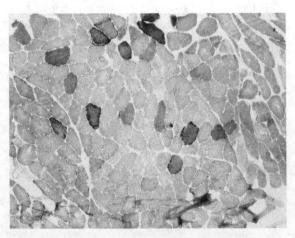

FIGURE 25-1 Combined cytochrome c oxidase (COX) and succinate dehydrogenase (SDH) staining of muscle tissue from the patient with a spastic-ataxia phenotype, demonstrating blue staining (displayed as black in this figure) COX negative-SDH positive fibers.

the finding of a thin corpus callosum on neuroimaging (e.g. SPG11 and SPG15). The *SPG7* gene is the first gene identified as a cause of autosomal recessive HSP (Casari et al., 1998). It encodes the paraplegin protein that is located in the inner mitochondrial membrane. Mutations in this gene often cause a complicated form of HSP, with clinical manifestations including cerebellar ataxia and cerebellar atrophy, optic atrophy, ptosis, chronic progressive external ophthalmoplegia-like features, and mitochondrial abnormalities on muscle biopsy (Klebe et al., 2012; van Gassen et al., 2012). There is now evidence to suggest that SPG7 is a disorder of mitochondrial DNA maintenance (Pfeffer et al., 2014).

The patient from the clinical vignette appeared to have an autosomal recessive condition given that several family members from a single generation were affected. He was investigated with a targeted next generation sequencing panel that allowed us to screen 10 well-established genes known to cause autosomal recessive HSP (as previously reported; Kumar et al., 2013). The autosomal recessive panel included the *CYP7B1, SPG7, SPG11, ZFYVE26, SPG20, SPG21/ACP33, FA2H, PNPLA6* and *GJC2* genes. The patient was found to be compound heterozygous for *SPG7* mutations, with a common mutation of known pathogenicity (p.A510V) and a novel mutation (p.S576W).

The patient was given appropriate genetic counseling and referred back to his clinician for ongoing management. Currently, there are no treatments to address the underlying neurodegenerative process. However, medications such as baclofen and intramuscular botulinum toxin injections may improve symptoms related to spasticity.

KEY POINTS TO REMEMBER ABOUT HEREDITARY SPASTIC PARAPLEGIA

- In "pure" forms of HSP, the chief clinical feature is spasticity in the lower limbs.
- In "complicated" forms of HSP, additional clinical features are present, such as cerebellar signs, ophthalmoplegia, ptosis, cognitive impairment, seizures, dysarthria, and peripheral neuropathy.

- There is marked genetic heterogeneity in HSP with at least 54 genes and 72 loci identified thus far.
- Mutations in *SPAST* (SPG4) are the most common cause of autosomal dominant forms of HSP.
- Mutations in *SPG7* (SPG7) can cause autosomal recessive HSP, which is frequently complicated by additional clinical findings including cerebellar ataxia, a chronic progressive external ophthalmoplegia-like phenotype, and changes consistent with mitochondrial dysfunction on muscle biopsy.

Further Reading

Casari, G., De Fusco, M., Ciarmatori, S., Zeviani, M., Mora, M., Fernandez, P., . . . & Ballabio, A. (1998). Spastic paraplegia and OXPHOS impairment caused by mutations in paraplegin, a nuclear-encoded mitochondrial metalloprotease. *Cell*, *93*, 973–983.

Finsterer, J., Loscher, W., Quasthoff, S., Wanschitz, J., Auer-Grumbach, M., & Stevanin, G. (2012). Hereditary spastic paraplegias with autosomal dominant, recessive, X-linked, or maternal trait of inheritance. *Journal of the Neurological Sciences*, *318*, 1–18.

Klebe, S., Depienne, C., Gerber, S., Challe, G., Anheim, M., Charles, P., . . . & Durr, A. (2012). Spastic paraplegia gene 7 in patients with spasticity and/or optic neuropathy. *Brain: A Journal of Neurology*, *135*, 2980–2993.

Kumar, K. R., Blair, N. F., Vandebona, H., Liang, C., Ng, K., Sharpe, D. M., . . . & Sue, C. M. (2013). Targeted next generation sequencing in SPAST-negative hereditary spastic paraplegia. *Journal of Neurology*.

Novarino, G., Fenstermaker, A. G., Zaki, M. S., Hofree, M., Silhavy, J. L., Heiberg, A. D., . . . & Gleeson, J. G. (2014) Exome sequencing links corticospinal motor neuron disease to common neurodegenerative disorders. *Science*, *343*, 506–511.

Pfeffer, G., Gorman, G. S., Griffin, H., Kurzawa-Akanbi, M., Blakely, E. L., Wilson, I., . . . & Chinnery, P. F. (2014) Mutations in the SPG7 gene cause chronic progressive external ophthalmoplegia through disordered mitochondrial DNA maintenance. *Brain: A Journal of Neurology*, Epub ahead of print.

Vandebona, H., Kerr, N. P., Liang, C., & Sue, C. M. (2012). SPAST mutations in Australian patients with hereditary spastic paraplegia. *Internal Medicine Journal*, *42*, 1342–1347.

van Gassen, K. L., van der Heijden, C. D., de Bot, S. T., den Dunnen, W. F., van den Berg, L. H., Verschuuren-Bemelmans, C. C., . . . & van de Warrenburg, B. P. (2012). Genotype-phenotype correlations in spastic paraplegia type 7: A study in a large Dutch cohort. *Brain: A Journal of Neurology*, *135*, 2994–3004

26 Inherited Prion Diseases

A 47-year-old man presents with a history of an unsteady gait, unpleasant burning and tingling sensations in both legs, and slurred speech. The symptoms have gradually developed over the last 2 years. Due to his leg problems, he had previously consulted an orthopedic surgeon who diagnosed lumbar spinal canal stenosis and suggested surgical treatment. The patient now seeks a second opinion. There was no past medical history of note, but the patient volunteered that his mother had died in her 60s because of dementia, and his maternal uncle died in his late 50s due to an unclear neurological condition causing gait and balance problems and later severe confusion.

On examination, the neuropsychiatric assessment was normal. Visual pursuit was saccadic and fixation suppression of the vestibular-ocular reflex (VOR) was incomplete.

There was muscle weakness (4 out of 5) in proximal leg muscles and areflexia but no muscle wasting. Babinski sign was negative. Light touch perception and vibration sense were preserved, but the patient reported painful dysesthesia in his legs, which increased during touch and did not correspond to a dermatomal distribution. He had very mild if any upper limb dysmetria but moderate to marked truncal ataxia and leg dysmetria. His gait was wide-based, unsteady, and slow. His speech was dysarthric.

What do you do now?

The patient has a clinical phenotype characterized by truncal and lower limb ataxia associated with sensory symptoms, which should be interpreted in the light of a positive family history suggesting autosomal dominant inheritance. Given the adult onset and chronic evolution of symptoms, autosomal dominant spinocerebellar ataxias (SCA) are top on the list of differential diagnoses. However, almost complete sparing of the arms and absent reflexes would be unusual for this group of disorders.

To better understand the nature of the dysesthesia, additional electrodiagnostic studies were performed, particularly since a number of SCAs can be associated with a peripheral neuropathy. In spite of severe sensory symptoms, motor and sensory nerve conduction studies were normal in this case. However, somatosensory evoked potentials (SEPs) showed slightly increased latencies after tibial nerve stimulation. The SEPs after median nerve stimulation were normal.

The combination of sensory symptoms, areflexia, and electrodiagnostic findings would be in favor of a posterior horn lesion but not a sensory neuropathy. Magnetic resonance imaging (MRI) of the brain and spinal cord and electroencephalography (EEG) were normal. The cerebrospinal fluid (CSF) was acellular with normal protein and glucose levels, although the 14-3-3 protein was positive and S100B protein was elevated.

In view of the positive family history, the clinical syndrome, and the results of additional investigations, familial prion disease was suspected. Genetic testing was initiated showing the P102L mutation in the human *prion protein* (*PRNP*) gene. This is in keeping with the diagnosis of Gerstmann-Sträussler-Scheinker syndrome (GSS), an inherited prion disease.

Human Prion Disease

Human prion diseases can be classified into sporadic, acquired, and inherited forms with Creutzfeldt-Jakob disease (CJD), Kuru, and GSS being classical examples.

Sporadic CJD is a rapidly progressive, multifocal dementia often associated with stimulus-sensitive myoclonus. Onset is usually in the 45- to 75-year age group. The disease progresses rapidly over weeks to akinetic mutism and death often within 2–3 months. Frequent additional neurological signs include parkinsonism, apraxia, cortical blindness, cerebellar ataxia, and pyramidal signs.

Kuru occurred in defined populations in the Eastern Highlands of Papua New Guinea. It was transmitted when relatives consumed the brain and internal organs of their deceased family members. The epidemic is thought to have originated after the consumption of a brain from an individual with sporadic CJD, given that sporadic CJD is known to occur at random in all populations.

Inherited prion disease accounts for around 15% of all human prion disease. The classical examples include GSS presenting as a chronic cerebellar ataxia syndrome, with dementia occurring later in a much more prolonged clinical course compared to CJD and fatal familial insomnia. GSS was first associated with the P102L *PRNP* mutation, but it has now become clear that it can also be caused by other mutations.

Over 20 pathogenic mutations have been described in inherited prion disease in two groups: (1) point mutations resulting in amino acid substitutions in the prion protein (PrP), or production of a stop codon resulting in expression of a truncated PrP; and (2) insertions encoding additional integral copies of an octapeptide repeat present in a tandem array of five copies in the normal protein. All inherited prion diseases including GSS are autosomal dominant. Kindreds with inherited prion disease have been described with CJD and GSS phenotypes but also with a range of other neurodegenerative syndromes. Phenotypic variability in families is large, encompassing both CJD- and GSS-like cases as well as other syndromes. Progressive dementia, cerebellar ataxia, pyramidal signs, pseudobulbar and amyotrophic features, and movement disorders can occur in variable combinations.

Onset of GSS is typically in the fifth decade but it can range from the 30s to late 60s. The disease duration is seven months to several years. The most commonly occurring primary presenting features of GSS are shown in the Figure 26-1.

Parkinsonism and severe psychiatric symptoms such as personality changes, delusions, paranoia, and visual hallucinations are present in about 50% of patients. In contrast, myoclonus and seizures that are characteristic of sporadic CJD are less common. Also, chorea is not a typical sign in GSS. However, the clinical presentation can be quite heterogeneous. Although a

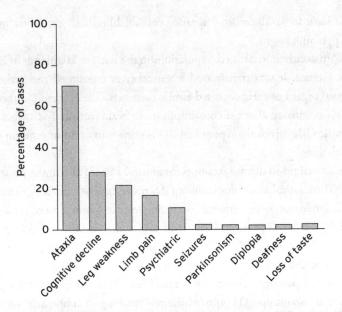

FIGURE 26-1 Relative frequency of symptoms and signs on presentation in GSS patients with the P102L mutation (Webb et al., 2008).

majority of patients present with the phenotype of progressive ataxia with a later onset of cognitive involvement, in a significant proportion psychiatric and cognitive features will dominate the early stages of the disease and can remain as the major clinical feature. A small group of GSS cases is characterized by a rapid and more global pattern of deficits reminiscent of sporadic CJD. Proximal leg weakness, areflexia, and sensory symptoms are present in the majority of patients. Interestingly, as suspected in this case on the basis of the electrodiagnostic studies, post mortem studies have shown severe involvement of the posterior horn in GSS patients.

Additional investigations can be helpful, and they typically show a pattern of abnormalities that differs from that of CJD. In most patients cell count and protein levels in CSF are normal. The 14-3-3 protein levels, however, are often, but not always, elevated. The EEG is usually normal or only shows nonspecific changes. In early stages, the MRI is often normal, and so typical signs associated with prion disease including the "pulvinar" sign, or cortical or basal ganglia signal abnormalities are usually absent. Some patients have multiple white matter lesions suggestive of vascular changes.

As the disease progresses, MRI may demonstrate cerebellar and generalized cerebral atrophy. Also, in the latter stages of the disease, DWI-, FLAIR-, or T2 weighted images can show signal abnormalities in the thalamus, caudate nucleus, frontal, occipital, or insular cortex similar to sporadic CJD.

KEY POINTS TO REMEMBER ABOUT INHERITED PRION DISEASES

- Inherited prion disease comprises about 15% of all human prion diseases.
- Gerstmann-Sträussler-Scheinker (GSS) disease is a classical autosomal dominant prion disease syndrome typically presenting with gait ataxia, later development of cognitive problems and a combination of lower leg weakness, dysesthesia, and areflexia.
- GSS is usually caused by the P102L *prion protein* (*PRNP*) mutation but can also be associated with many other *PRNP* mutations.
- The 14-3-3 levels in the CSF may be elevated and raise suspicion of a prion disease, although the findings of additional investigations, particularly brain imaging, are not specific for GSS or other inherited prion diseases.

Further Reading

Arata, H., Takashima, H., Hirano, R., Tomimitsu, H., Machigashira, K., Izumi, K., & Arimura, K. (2006). Early clinical signs and imaging findings in Gerstmann-Sträussler–Scheinker syndrome (Pro102Leu). *Neurology, 66*, 1672–1678.

Capellari, S., Strammiello, R., Saverioni, D., Kretzschmar, H., & Parchi, P. (2011). Genetic Creutzfeldt–Jakob disease and fatal familial insomnia: insights into phenotypic variability and disease pathogenesis. *Acta Neuropathologica, 121*, 21–37.

Collinge, J. (2001). Prion diseases of humans, animals: Their causes and molecular basis. *Annual Review of Neuroscience, 24*, 519–550.

Mead, S., Poulter, M., Beck, J., Webb, T. E., Campbell, T. A., Linehan, J. M.,...& Collinge, J. (2006). Inherited prion disease with six octapeptide repeat insertional mutation–molecular analysis of phenotypic heterogeneity. *Brain: A Journal of Neurology, 129*, 2297–2317.

Rusina, R., Fiala, J., Holada, K., Matějčková, M., Nováková, J., Ampapa, R.,...& Matěj, R. (2013). Gerstmann–Sträussler–Scheinker syndrome with the P102L pathogenic mutation presenting as familial Creutzfeldt–Jakob disease: A case report and review of the literature. *Neurocase, 19*, 41–53.

Webb, T. E., Poulter, M., Beck, J., Uphill, J., Adamson, G., Campbell, T., . . . & Mead, S. (2008). Phenotypic heterogeneity and genetic modification of P102L inherited prion disease in an international series. *Brain: A Journal of Neurology, 131*, 2632–2646.

Yamada, M., Tomimitsu, H., Yokota, T., Tomi, H., Sunohara, N., Mukoyama, M., . . . & Mizusawa, H. (1999). Involvement of the spinal posterior horn in Gerstmann–Straussler–Scheinker disease (PrP P102L). *Neurology, 52*, 260–265.

27 Frontotemporal Dementia— Amyotrophic Lateral Sclerosis Syndrome

You are referred a 45-year-old woman to the neurogenetics clinic with a progressive cognitive impairment.

Her problems started at the age of 41 years, when relatives noticed that she was no longer participating in conversations and was having trouble with her thinking. She had poor planning, was unable to budget, and had accumulated a large debt. She also developed urinary incontinence of which she was often unconcerned, and she refused to wear incontinence pads. She was no longer able to continue her work as a clerical officer. She eventually had to move in with a relative due to difficulties with hygiene, self-care, and preparing and eating meals. There was also problems with impulse control. For example, she would often rush to the phone in order to buy objects advertized on television. Relatives observed that her appetite had increased. Additionally, she would sometimes choke while eating food and her speech had become slurred. She also has trouble with activities requiring fine motor control such as doing up buttons, tying shoelaces, and writing.

Interestingly, the patient has a positive family history (Figure 27-1). Her brother (III.3), aged 39, had similar cognitive and behavioral problems, and was diagnosed with schizophrenia 10 years previously. Her only other sibling (III.2) was 42 years of age and was unaffected. Her mother (II.2) developed symptoms of motor neurone disease from the age of 38 years and died from complications of this illness at the age of 42 years. Her maternal grandfather (I.1) also died of motor neuron disease at the age of 45 years.

On examination, the patient was alert and attentive and reasonably engaged in the consultation, although she tended to speak only when asked questions. At one stage, she is interrupted half way through taking off her glasses, and she leaves them hanging from one ear. The glasses stayed crooked on her face while she continued to talk. When alerted to this, she pulled the glasses back over her ears but kept her hands on the handles of the glasses. She could only perform one cycle of the Luria three-step test before perseverating and losing the correct sequence. On cranial nerve examination, you observe the presence of square wave jerks, and her speech is slow and hesitant. There was no evidence of wasting or fasciculations of the tongue. Examination of the upper and lower limbs showed no wasting or fasciculations, and tone and power were normal, but there was generalized hyperreflexia. There was no evidence of primitive reflexes such as the glabellar or grasp reflex. However, she had difficulty mimicking gestures and finger postures with her left hand. Her gait was unsteady with a tendency to lean to the right, but her postural reflexes were preserved.

Nerve conduction studies and electromyography showed nonspecific changes only without fibrillations or fasciculations. Brain magnetic resonance imaging showed evidence of frontal and temporal lobe atrophy.

What do you do now?

The patient appears to have a phenotype in keeping with the behavioral variant of frontotemporal dementia (FTD), with a decline in executive and interpersonal skills, impulsive behaviors, apathy, inertia, and perseveration. The FTD spectrum overlaps with the syndromes of progressive supranuclear palsy, corticobasal syndrome, and FTD with amyotrophic lateral sclerosis (FTD-ALS; Warren, Rohrer, & Rosser, 2013). The patient's family history is suggestive of a FTD-ALS overlap syndrome with an autosomal dominant pattern of inheritance.

Three causative genes are responsible for over 80% of cases of FTD in families with a clear autosomal dominant family history: *MAPT, GRN*, and *C9ORF72* (Loy, Schofield, Turner, & Kwok, 2013). In addition to the three main FTD causing genes, there are many rarer genetic causes including mutations in the *VCP* (see chapter 24, this volume), *FUS,* and *CHMP2B* genes.

An abnormal expansion of a GGGGCC hexanucleotide repeat in a noncoding region of the *chromosome 9 open reading frame 72* gene (*C9ORF72*)

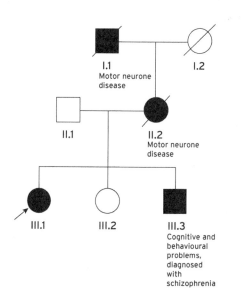

FIGURE 27-1 Pedigree of the family with frontotemporal dementia and amyotrophic lateral sclerosis. Males are represented by squares, females by circles. Filled symbols indicate affected family members. The index patient (III.1) is indicated with an arrow. A diagonal line through the symbol indicates a deceased family member.

is the most common genetic abnormality in familial and sporadic FTD and ALS, and is the cause in most families when both FTD and ALS are coinherited (Mackenzie, Frick, & Neumann, 2013). Furthermore, psychiatric symptoms occur frequently in the context of FTD-ALS due to *C9ORF72* expansions (Snowden et al., 2013). It is notable that the brother of the patient from the clinical vignette was diagnosed with schizophrenia, increasing your suspicion that this family has a *C9ORF72* mutation.

The patient was enrolled in a study in which patients with FTD were screened for the *C9ORF72* hexanucleotide repeat expansion using Southern blotting of genomic DNA, and she was identified as a mutation carrier (Patient 12, Dobson-Stone et al., 2013). You provide the patient and her family with genetic counseling and continue to see the patient in your clinic for symptomatic management.

KEY POINTS TO REMEMBER ABOUT GENETIC FORMS OF FRONTOTEMPORAL DEMENTIA-AMYOTROPHIC LATERAL SCLEROSIS SYNDROME

- The frontotemporal dementia (FTD) spectrum overlaps with the syndromes of progressive supranuclear palsy, corticobasal syndrome, and FTD with amyotrophic lateral sclerosis (FTD-ALS).
- Three causative genes are responsible for over 80% of cases of FTD in families with a clear autosomal dominant family history: *MAPT*, *GRN*, and *C9ORF72*.
- Rarer genetic causes of FTD include mutations in the *VCP*, *FUS*, and *CHMP2B* genes.
- An abnormal expansion of a hexanucleotide repeat in a noncoding region of the *C9ORF72* gene is the most common genetic abnormality in familial and sporadic FTD and ALS, and is the most common cause in families when both FTD and ALS are coinherited.
- The presence of psychiatric symptoms in the context of FTD-ALS should alert clinicians to the possibility of a *C9ORF72* expansion.

Further Reading

Dobson-Stone, C., Hallupp, M., Loy, C. T., Thompson, E. M., Haan, E., Sue, C.M.,...& Kwok, J. B. (2013). C9ORF72 repeat expansion in Australian and Spanish frontotemporal dementia patients. *PloS One 8*:e56899.

Loy, C. T., Schofield, P. R., Turner, A. M., & Kwok, J. B. (2014). Genetics of dementia. *Lancet, 383*, 828–840.

Mackenzie, I. R., Frick, P., & Neumann, M. (2014). The neuropathology associated with repeat expansions in the C9ORF72 gene. *Acta neuropathologica, 127*, 347–357.

Snowden, J. S., Harris, J., Richardson, A., Rollinson, S., Thompson, J. C., Neary, D.,...& Pickering-Brown, S. (2013). Frontotemporal dementia with amyotrophic lateral sclerosis: a clinical comparison of patients with and without repeat expansions in C9orf72. *Amyotrophic Lateral Sclerosis & Frontotemporal Degeneration, 14*, 172–176.

Warren, J. D., Rohrer, J. D., & Rossor, M. N. (2013). Clinical review. Frontotemporal dementia. *British Medical Journal, 347*, f4827.

28 Neurodegeneration with Brain Iron Accumulation

A mother brings her 20-year-old daughter with severe cognitive and behavioral deficits to the neurology outpatient clinic for a third opinion because of an unclear diagnosis. She reports that after a normal delivery, impaired psychomotor development was noted in the first year of life. She only began to walk by the age of 3 years, indicating a marked delay in her motor milestones. She remained clumsy but developed a limited repertoire of goal-directed movements. Hand movements and coordination never fully developed. She was able to articulate a few words, but these were difficult to discern. Often during the day she would engage in repetitive hand wringing and clapping movements and repeat single words or word fragments. The patient's mother described her as even-tempered, quiet, and shy. Over the last two years, her walking ability has deteriorated further, she has begun to fall frequently, and has developed a stooped posture. Previous investigations had been normal apart from unclear signal changes in the basal ganglia on magnetic resonance imaging (MRI). There was no family history of note.

On examination, she is initially shy and withdrawn with very limited eye contact, but she starts to interact with you after a while. She follows simple commands. Upward gaze is somewhat limited but eye movements are otherwise normal. There is mild spasticity in the arms and legs with brisk reflexes, but plantar responses are flexor. There is mild dystonic posturing of both arms and an unusual posture of both feet with slight plantar flexion and marked eversion. Her arm movements are bradykinetic. There is severe axial hypokinesia. Frequently, there are hand-clapping stereotypies. She walks slowly with bent knees, a markedly stooped posture and small steps. Her postural stability is impaired.

In summary, this young woman presents with severe psychomotor developmental delay, parkinsonism, mild generalized spasticity, dystonia, and a possible vertical-gaze palsy.

What do you do now?

There are a number of clinical signs but no single one is diagnostic. Given the early onset of spasticity and dystonia in the first year of life, cerebral palsy should be considered, although the development of pronounced parkinsonism and the progressive nature of the illness argue against this diagnosis. A disease belonging to the group of disorders with disturbed dopamine biosynthesis or neurotransmission is a possibility, but in these conditions parkinsonism usually starts earlier and is not associated with brain MRI abnormalities, as in this patient. Parkinsonism plus dystonia could be indicative of one of the complex dystonias due to neurodegeneration including Huntington disease or Niemann-Pick type C. A thorough review of the MRI images would be helpful to distinguish these conditions and should be the next step (Figure 28-1).

The MRI is suggestive of iron deposition in the globus pallidus and substantia nigra. A computerized tomography (CT) scan of the head was normal, excluding the possibility of basal ganglia calcification and thus confirming your suspicion of a disorder of iron metabolism.

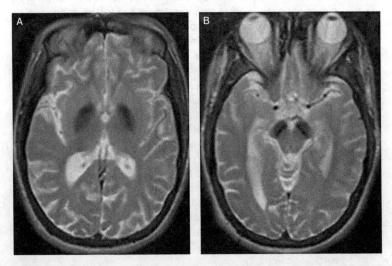

FIGURE 28-1 MRI of the patient showing signal abnormalities in the globus pallidus (A) and substantia nigra (B). Both structures are hypointense on axial T2 sequences indicating high levels of iron.

The Spectrum of Neurodegeneration with Brain Iron Accumulation Disorders

Neurodegeneration with brain iron accumulation (NBIA) encompasses a group of progressive disorders characterized by excessive iron deposition in the brain. Almost all patients with NBIA have abnormal iron accumulation in the basal ganglia, which is reflected in hypointense lesions that are predominantly but not exclusively located in the globus pallidus. Some disorders are also associated with iron accumulation in the substantia nigra pars reticulata and other imaging features such as cerebral, cerebellar, and brainstem atrophy. The distribution of iron deposition and patterns of associated signs are often, but not always, characteristic for a certain disease, as will be discussed later.

The best known form of NBIA, autosomal recessive pantothenate kinase associated neurodegeneration, or PKAN, is caused by mutations in the *PANK2* gene, and currently accounts for approximately 50% of identified cases of NBIA. This percentage is likely to decrease as new entities with unknown prevalence belonging to the NBAI family are being recognized. Many NBAI cases have probably been overlooked in the past.

In classic PKAN, onset is early, usually before 6 years of age, and progression is rapid. Affected children often present with dystonic gait, dysarthria, and limb rigidity. Corticospinal tract involvement causes additional spasticity. Developmental delay and attention deficit hyperactivity disorder are also common. In PKAN, a central region of hyperintensity in the globus pallidus with surrounding hypointensity on T2-weighted images is pathognomonic for this disease. This so called "eye-of-the-tiger" sign (Figure 28-2) is often found in patients with mutations in the *PANK2* gene.

Given that there was no "eye-of-the-tiger" sign in our patient, a diagnosis of PKAN is unlikely. A key feature was iron deposition in the substantia nigra. Of late, this sign has been found in patients with either mitochondrial membrane protein-associated neurodegeneration (MPAN) or beta-propeller protein-associated neurodegeneration (BPAN).

Autosomal recessive MPAN is caused by mutations in the *C19orf12* gene, leading to NBIA and prominent, widespread Lewy body pathology (Hogarth, et al.). It is characterized by limb and occasionally generalized dystonia, parkinsonism (with varying combinations of bradykinesia, rigidity, tremor, and postural instability), cognitive decline progressing to dementia, prominent neuropsychiatric abnormalities, and motor neuronopathy. Iron

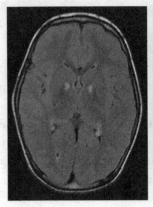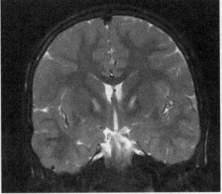

FIGURE 28-2 MRI of a patient with pantothenate kinase-associated neurodegeneration demonstrating signal abnormalities in the globus pallidus on axial FLAIR (left panel) and coronal T2 (right panel) sequences. More central areas of hyperintensity surrounded by peripheral hypointensity in the globus pallidus are very characteristic for this disease.

accumulates in the substantia nigra and globus pallidus as in the case under discussion. However, there is often a unique T2-hyperintense streaking between the hypointense internal and external globus pallidus, which was not present in our patient. Also, there was no prominent muscle wasting, arguing against a motor neuronopathy.

X-linked dominant beta-propeller protein-associated neurodegeneration (BPAN) is associated with mutations in the *WDR45* gene. The *WDR45* gene was sequenced in the patient from the clinical vignette, and she was found to have a heterozygous mutation in intron 8 (c.519+1_519+3delGTG, recently reported by Ichinose et al.), consistent with the diagnosis of BPAN.

BPAN is the first X-linked disorder in the NBAI family (Hayflick et al., 2013). Most patients are female. To date, all mutations are known or suspected to arise de novo, and males are predicted or known to harbor postzygotic mutations explaining their viability. Similar to Rett syndrome, another X-linked dominant disorder caused by mutations in the *MECP2* gene (Temudo et al., 2008), female patients may harbor either germline or somatic mutations. If their mutation is present in germ cells, then 50% of female offspring will have BPAN, and 50% of male offspring will probably not survive. Parental testing for *WDR45* gene mutations should be performed because very mildly affected individuals with a low level of somatic mosaicism or "favorable" skewing of X chromosome inactivation may be at high risk for having a severely affected child. Genetic testing of *WDR45* is now widely available in the clinical setting. Diagnostic testing of multiple tissues may be necessary to identify mutations in *WDR45* in those with somatic mosaicism.

BPAN has a characteristic phenotype with global developmental delay and slow language and motor gains in early childhood until adolescence or early adulthood, when dystonia, parkinsonism, and cognitive decline become manifest. Autism, seizures, spasticity, disordered sleep, and stereotypies are also common in childhood. Levodopa can considerably improve parkinsonian features but, unfortunately, dyskinesias develop in many patients. On neuroimaging, iron appears to accumulate first in the substantia nigra and later in globus pallidus. A distinguishing and possibly unique feature of BPAN is a bright halo on T1-weighted imaging in the substantia nigra and cerebral peduncles present in many patients. In keeping with brain imaging, post mortem investigations show that changes in substantia nigra dominate those found in globus pallidus. Cases of BPAN have previously been labeled as static encephalopathy with neurodegeneration in adulthood (SENDA), but this term is no longer favored.

BPAN has some similarities with atypical Rett syndrome. Both BPAN and atypical Rett syndrome cause neurodevelopmental regression with loss of previously acquired skills, autism, and are associated with atypical stereotypies and the development of parkinsonism. Both conditions are X-linked dominant, which is a rare pattern of inheritance. Therefore, *WDR45* should be added to the growing list of genes associated with a Rett-like phenotype.

Other diseases in the NBAI family include autosomal recessive infantile neuroaxonal dystrophy (INAD) and atypical neuroaxonal dystrophy (NAD), idiopathic NBAI, fatty acid hydroxylase-associated neurodegeneration (FAHN), and neuroferritinopathy.

INAD and NAD are caused by mutations in the *PLA2G6* gene and also exhibit high brain iron in about half of cases (Gregory et al., 2009). Progressive dystonia, dysarthria, and behavioral abnormalities including hyperactivity and impulsivity are common in NAD and have an onset around the age of 4 years. Mutations in the *PLA2G6* gene can also cause the syndrome of juvenile parkinsonism associated with pyramidal signs, dementia, psychiatric features, and cerebral as well as cerebellar atrophy without brain iron accumulation on MRI (Paisan-Ruiz et al., 2009).

The clinical spectrum of idiopathic NBIA is broad. However, most affected patients have progressive dystonia, rigidity and dysarthria, and optic atrophy is present in many cases. Developmental delay or cognitive impairment are more frequent in this group than in PKAN. Age at onset and progression vary greatly.

In autosomal recessive FAHN, which is due to mutations in the FA2H gene (Kruer et al., 2010), patients present with spastic tetraparesis, ataxia, and generalized dystonia with onset in childhood and episodic neurological decline. Neuroimaging typically demonstrates T2 hypointensity in the globus pallidus, confluent T2 white matter hyperintensities, and profound pontocerebellar atrophy.

Neuroferritinopathy is an autosomal dominant adult-onset disorder caused by mutation in the *FTL* gene (Curtis et al., 2001; Crompton et al., 2005). It presents with progressive adult-onset chorea or dystonia and subtle cognitive deficits. Many affected patients develop a characteristic orofacial action-specific dystonia induced by speech leading to dysarthrophonia. Frontalis overactivity, orolingual dyskinesia, and dysphagia are also common. MRI often shows cystic lesions in the basal ganglia and bilateral pallidal necrosis, in addition to iron accumulation in the caudate, globus pallidus, putamen, substantia nigra, and red nuclei.

KEY POINTS TO REMEMBER ABOUT NEURODEGENERATION WITH BRAIN IRON ACCUMULATION

- Neurodegeneration with brain iron accumulation (NBAI) is a large and growing group of heterogeneous disorders typically starting in childhood with variable combinations of developmental delay, dystonia, and parkinsonism.
- Abnormal iron deposition on MRI is a hallmark of most diseases in the NBAI spectrum with the globus pallidus and substantia nigra typically being affected. The distribution of iron accumulation and additional imaging patterns are often distinct.
- The mode of inheritance can be autosomal recessive, autosomal dominant, or X-linked dominant.
- Beta-propeller protein-associated neurodegeneration (BPAN) caused by *WDR45* gene mutations should be considered in all *MECP2* mutation-negative patients with a Rett-like phenotype.

Further Reading

Crompton, D. E., Chinnery, P. F., Bates, D., Walls, T. J., Jackson, M. J., Curtis, A. J., & Burns, J. (2005). Spectrum of movement disorders in neuroferritinopathy. *Movement Disorders, 20,* 95–99.

Curtis, A. R., Fey, C., Morris, C. M., Bindoff, L. A., Ince, P. G., Chinnery, P. F.,... & Burn, J. (2001). Mutation in the gene encoding ferritin light polypeptide causes dominant adult-onset basal ganglia disease. *Nature Genetics, 28,* 350–354.

Gregory, A., Polster, B. J., & Hayflick, S. J. (2009). Clinical and genetic delineation of neurodegeneration with brain iron accumulation. *Journal of Medical Genetics, 46,* 73–80.

Hayflick, S. J., Kruer, M. C., Gregory, A., Haack, T. B., Kurian, M. A., Houlden, H. H.,... & Hogarth, P. (2013). β-propeller protein-associated neurodegeneration: a new X-linked dominant disorder with brain iron accumulation. *Brain: A Journal of Neurology, 136,* 1708–1717.

Hogarth, P., Gregory, A., Kruer, M. C., Sanford, L., Wagoner, W., Natowicz, M. R.,... & Hayflick, S. J. (2013). New NBIA subtype: Genetic, clinical, pathologic, and radiographic features of MPAN. *Neurology, 80,* 268–275.

Inchinose, Y., Miwa, M., Onohara, A., Obi, K., Shindo, K., Saitsu, H.,... & Takiyama, Y. (2013). Characteristic MRI findings in beta-propeller protein associated neurodegeneration (BPAN). *Neurology in Clinical Practice, Epub ahead of print.* doi:10.1212/01. CPJ.0000437694.17888.9b

Kruer, M. C., Paisán-Ruiz, C., Boddaert, N., Yoon, M. Y., Hama, H., Gregory, A.,... & Hayflick, S. J. (2010). Defective FA2H leads to a novel form of neurodegeneration with brain iron accumulation (NBIA). *Annals of Neurology, 68,* 611–618.

Paisan-Ruiz, C., Bhatia, K. P., Li, A., Hernandez, D., Davis, M., Wood, N. W.,... & Schneider, S. A. (2009). Characterization of PLA2G6 as a locus for dystonia-parkinsonism. *Annals of Neurology, 65,* 19–23.

Temudo, T., Ramos, E., Dias, K., Barbot, C., Vieira, J. P., Moreira, A.,... & Maciel, P. (2008). Movement disorders in Rett syndrome: an analysis of 60 patients with detected MECP2 mutation and correlation with mutation type. *Movement Disorders, 23,* 1384–1390.

29 Coincidental Occurrence of Two Monogenic Disorders

A 10-year-old boy with myotonic dystrophy (see chapter 21, this volume) is referred to your movement disorders clinic because of slowly progressive ataxia since the age of 9 years. First signs of the myotonic dystrophy had become apparent at 4 years of age, as he started developing cramps when holding small objects. The patient then went on to develop the typical clinical picture of myotonic dystrophy including slowly progressive generalized weakness. His family history was strongly suggestive of dominant inheritance of the condition, and repeat expansions in the *DMPK* gene (300–400 repeats in both alleles) genetically confirmed the clinical diagnosis of myotonic dystrophy type 1.

On examination, the patient showed a complex neurological syndrome of a myotonic facies, saccadic pursuit, gaze-evoked nystagmus, dysmetria, gait ataxia, generalized muscle weakness, contraction and percussion myotonia, loss of deep tendon reflexes, and impaired proprioception and vibration sense.

What do you do now?

Although the patient exhibits typical signs of the myotonic dystrophy, he also has additional neurological signs of a generalized cerebellar syndrome that are outside the usual phenotypic spectrum of the initially diagnosed genetic condition. As the ataxia is slowly progressive, you suspect that the patient may also suffer from a second, potentially inherited condition. Since his family history is negative for ataxia and the age at onset is early, you order a genetic test for Friedreich ataxia, the most common known form of recessive ataxia. Testing for repeat expansions in the *FXN* gene reveals 500–900 repeats in both alleles, thereby confirming a second neurogenetic condition in the same patient.

You carefully assess the patient for possible concomitant feature of Friedrich ataxia including diabetes mellitus, vision and hearing impairment, and particularly cardiac involvement, which is present in most patients with Friedreich ataxia. Importantly, the heart is also commonly involved in myotonic dystrophy, and the patient's father had died from a cardiac arrhythmia. Treatment of both the myotonic dystrophy and the Friedrich ataxia is symptomatic with physiotherapy playing an important role. You continue to closely monitor the patient in your clinic and you counsel the family with respect to the coincidence of two severe neurogenetic conditions and the likely poor prognosis.

Although co-occurrence of mutations in more than one gene in the same patient is rare, such a finding is statistically more likely than previously thought. One of the remarkable discoveries of the 1,000 Genomes Project is that each person carries an average of 50–100 loss-of-function variants previously implicated in inherited diseases (Abecasis et al., 2010). With >1,000 known neurogenetic conditions, it becomes increasingly conceivable that individuals even from outbred populations may inherit more than one pathogenic mutation. Thus, in cases of an unusually "broad phenotypic spectrum," an independent cause of the additional signs should be considered, because this may greatly impact the management and counseling of the patient.

KEY POINTS TO REMEMBER ABOUT THE COINCIDENTAL OCCURRENCE OF TWO MONOGENIC DISORDERS

- If a patient has additional neurological signs outside the usual phenotypic spectrum of the initially diagnosed genetic condition, you should consider the presence of a possible independent cause, which may also have Mendelian inheritance.
- As demonstrated by the 1,000 Genomes Project, which found that each person carries an average of 50–100 loss-of-function variants previously implicated in inherited diseases, co-occurrence of two neurogenetic conditions in the same patient is more common and statistically more likely than previously thought.
- Although a gene test is often considered as "gold standard" for establishing a diagnosis, careful clinical observation and reasoning beyond the results of a genetic test remain highly important.
- Establishing more than one neurogenetic condition in the same individual impacts clinical management and genetic counseling.

Further Reading

Abecasis, G. R., Altshuler, D., Auton, A., Brooks, L. D., Durbin, R. M., Gibbs, R. A.,...& McVean, G. A. (2010). A map of human genome variation from population-scale sequencing. *Nature*, 467(7319), 1061–1073.

30 Direct-to-Consumer Genetic Testing

A 55-year-old teacher was given a health-related personal genetics service kit for his birthday and recently obtained the results of this genetic analysis from a private company via the Internet. Although his direct-to-consumer genetic testing (DTCGT) revealed an average risk for most of the investigated conditions, an increased risk for Parkinson disease (PD) was predicted based on certain gene variants. The customer consulted a neurologist who did not detect any signs of PD and reassured him that there was currently no reason to believe that he might be developing PD. However, the man remained anxious about his reported increased risk for PD and seeks additional advice at your neurogenetics clinic.

What do you do now?

You reiterate that the man is currently free of any signs of PD and thus a diagnosis of PD can be ruled out at this point in time. However, you also mention that you cannot completely exclude the possibility that he might develop PD in the future. PD is a late-onset disease with an average of onset in the late 50s to early 60s, with a number of known risk factors, of which ageing and a positive family history are the most important ones. After having ruled out by history that any other family member has suffered from PD, you carefully study the report from the genetic testing company. Usually, information is not only given for "risk variants" (common genetic polymorphisms that may increase the risk to develop a certain disease) but also for selected mutations in genes causing monogenic forms of the disease. One such example is the p.G2019S mutation in the *LRRK2* gene, which is the most common known genetic cause of PD (see chapter 6, this volume). Importantly, this mutation is sufficient to cause PD in an age-dependent manner. As our DTCGT customer is negative for this mutation, you explain to him that he is not a carrier of this common mutation, which would confer a very high genetic risk. You also mention, however, that not all known genetic causes of PD were covered by the panel offered by the DTCGT company and, thus, although very unlikely, the presence of a rare monogenic cause of PD cannot be ruled out based on the results of the test.

Regarding the "increased genetic risk" for PD, you explain to the patient that a number of common genetic variants, also found at considerable frequencies in the general population, have been found to be associated with a higher risk of PD. However, even if several of these risk variants happen to coincide, the risk to develop PD will only be increased 2.5-fold (Nalls et al., 2011). Given the PD prevalence of 0.14% in the general population, the corresponding lifetime risk for our DTCGT customer seeking advice would still be as low as 0.35% (Klein & Ziegler, 2011). You reassure him that this is a very small overall risk and that the only advice you have for his him is to continue leading his healthy lifestyle.

DTCGT has enabled individuals to purchase genetic tests and receive results without the intervention of a health professional. Shortly after DTCGT became available, the American Society of Human Genetics provided a statement on DTCGT. The first recommendation reads as follows: "Companies offering DTCGT should disclose the sensitivity, specificity, and predictive value of the test, and the populations for which this information is known, in a readily understandable and accessible fashion" (Hudson et al., 2007). However, even if provided in a transparent fashion, it is difficult for most individuals and even for many doctors to adequately interpret the risk assessment. As in our case, the results of the genetic analysis can cause considerable uncertainty and anxiety, requiring extensive posttest counseling. According to a recent systematic review, the authors of position statements, policies, and recommendations described more potential harms than benefits. Some authors stated that direct-to-consumer testing should be actively discouraged, whereas others supported consumer rights to make autonomous choices (Skirton et al., 2012). Notably, large companies providing DTCGT have currently suspended their health-related genetic tests to comply with the U.S. Food and Drug Administration's directive to discontinue new consumer access until they can provide satisfactory evidence that the results are reliable and will not jeopardize consumers' health.

KEY POINTS TO REMEMBER ABOUT DIRECT-TO-CONSUMER GENETIC TESTING

- Direct-to-consumer genetic testing (DTCGT) has enabled individuals to purchase genetic tests and receive results without the intervention of a health professional.
- Although selected monogenic diseases are covered by these panels, the majority of the information provided usually concerns an assessment of risk to develop various common diseases. In many cases, this information is not easy to interpret for the customers and sometimes even for their doctors.
- A report of an "increased risk" to develop a certain disease, such as Parkinson disease (PD), may cause considerable uncertainty and anxiety, which can be reduced by careful posttest genetic counseling. For example, even if the risk to develop PD is increased 2.5-fold, the lifetime risk for PD may be as low as 0.35%.
- The U.S. Food and Drug Administration has recently issued a directive to DTCGT companies to discontinue new consumer access to DTCGT until satisfactory evidence is provided that the results are reliable and will not jeopardize consumers' health.

Further Reading

Hudson, K., Javitt, G., Burke, W., & Byers, P. (2007). ASHG Statement* on direct-to-consumer genetic testing in the United States. *Obstetrics & Gynecology*, *110*(6), 1392–1395.

Klein, C., & Ziegler, A. (2011). From GWAS to clinical utility in Parkinson's disease. *Lancet*, *377*(9766), 613–614.

Nalls, M. A., Plagnol, V., Hernandez, D. G., Sharma, M., Sheerin, U. M., Saad, M.,... & Wood, N. W. (2011). Imputation of sequence variants for identification of genetic risks for Parkinson's disease: A meta-analysis of genome-wide association studies. *Lancet*, *377*(9766), 641–649.

Skirton, H., Goldsmith, L., Jackson, L., & O'Connor, A. (2012). Direct to consumer genetic testing: a systematic review of position statements, policies and recommendations. *Clinical Genetics*, *82*(3), 210–218.

31 Incidental Findings in Genetic Testing

A five-year-old boy of Kurdish extraction is referred to your neurogenetics clinic for evaluation of mental retardation. He is the first child of reportedly unrelated parents and was born after an uneventful pregnancy and delivery. He had a normal karyotype. He underwent array comparative genomic hybridization (aCGH) to test for copy number variations (gains or losses of a portion of a chromosome) that might account for his mental retardation, as described previously (Netzer et al., 2009). Although the test results were uninformative regarding the possible cause of his mental retardation, they unexpectedly revealed a deletion spanning exons 4 and 5 of the *Parkin* gene. The parents plan to have another child and ask you about the risk for their son to develop Parkinson disease (PD) and for any future child to inherit the *Parkin* deletion.

What do you do now?

You must first validate the results of the aCGH analysis by quantitative PCR (qPCR) or by multiplex ligation-dependent probe amplification (MLPA), which is commercially offered by most genetic testing laboratories. After confirmation of the exon deletion in *Parkin* and in response to the parents' request to clarify the situation, you offer testing for this mutation to the parents in order to determine whether the mutation is inherited from one of the parents or whether it has arisen de novo in the son. As the parents are both unaffected, this test requires pre- and posttest counseling by a human geneticist or authorized specialist/genetic counselor. Molecular analysis revealed that the *Parkin* mutation was inherited from the mother.

As Parkin-linked PD is transmitted in an autosomal recessive fashion, a second mutated allele would be required to cause disease. As MLPA is only able to detect gene dosage changes (deletions or duplications of whole exons) but is not a qualitative method, you proceed to sequencing of the parental DNA for other mutations in the *Parkin* gene, such as point mutations or small deletions or insertions. As the index patient is a 5-year-old minor and unaffected by parkinsonism, testing of the child's DNA is not indicated. Sequence analysis of the *Parkin* gene of both parents does not reveal any additional mutation(s).

HOW DO YOU COUNSEL THE FAMILY?

You explain to the parents that the *Parkin* deletion in their son is an incidental finding that does not explain his mental retardation. Furthermore, this mutation is highly unlikely to result in PD, as it is present in the heterozygous state only. Notably, there is an ongoing debate about whether heterozygous *Parkin* mutations may serve as a risk factor for late-onset PD (Klein et al., 2007; Sharp et al., 2013); however, if present, this risk is likely to be very small in an individual mutation carrier, especially when considering that heterozygous *Parkin* mutations occur at a frequency of 1–3% in the normal population (Brüggemann et al., 2009). Thus, the risk for the mother to develop PD is likewise negligible. Any future offspring of the parents will be at 50% risk of inheriting the *Parkin* deletion from his or her mother. You also assure the family that no special treatment or lifestyle is recommended (or available) for carriers of a heterozygous *Parkin* mutation. The presence of a mutation in the heterozygous state may only become potentially relevant when their children start family planning. As the family originates from a population in which consanguineous marriages are relatively common, the possibility of two heterozygous mutations coming together may have to be considered.

Incidental findings are previously undiagnosed genetic findings or conditions that are discovered unintentionally and are unrelated to the current medical problem, in this case the patient's mental retardation. Given the rapid technological advances in molecular genetics, incidental findings by aGCH or by exome and genome sequencing (sequence analysis of all coding regions of the genome or of the entire genome, respectively) are becoming increasingly common. The American College of Medical Genetics and Genomics (ACMG) recently published a policy statement on clinical molecular analysis emphasizing the importance of alerting the patient/family to the possibility of such results in pretest counseling discussions as well as reporting of results (Green et al., 2013).

Given that a heterozygous *Parkin* deletion is highly unlikely to cause PD and potential preventive measures are currently unavailable, no additional action is required in this case, apart from the detailed counseling of the family. There are, however, a number of genetic conditions that are either treatable or even preventable. The ACMG provides a list of such conditions, genes, and variants recommended for return of incidental findings (Green et al., 2013).

KEY POINTS TO REMEMBER ABOUT INCIDENTAL FINDINGS IN GENETIC TESTING

- Incidental findings are previously undiagnosed genetic findings or conditions that are discovered unintentionally and are unrelated to the current medical problem.
- Given the rapid technological advances in molecular genetics, incidental findings by exome and genome sequencing (sequence analysis of all coding regions of the genome or of the entire genome, respectively) or by array comparative genomic hybridization are becoming increasingly common.
- The American College of Medical Genetics and Genomics (ACMG) recently published a policy statement on clinical molecular analysis emphasizing the importance of alerting the patient/family to the possibility of such results in pretest counseling discussions as well as reporting of results.

Further Reading

Brüggemann, N., Mitterer, M., Lanthaler, A. J., Djarmati, A., Hagenah, J., Wiegers, K.,...& Lohmann, K. (2009). Frequency of heterozygous Parkin mutations in healthy subjects: need for careful prospective follow-up examination of mutation carriers. *Parkinsonism Related Disorders, 15*(6), 425–429.

Green, R. C., Berg, J. S., Grody, W. W., Kalia, S. S., Korf, B. R., Martin, C. L.,...& Biesecker, L. G. (2013). ACMG recommendations for reporting of incidental findings in clinical exome and genome sequencing. *Genetics in Medicine, 15*(7), 565–574.

Klein, C., Lohmann-Hedrich, K., Rogaeva, E., Schlossmacher, M. G., & Lang, A. E. (2007). Deciphering the role of heterozygous mutations in genes associated with parkinsonism. *Lancet Neurology, 6*(7), 652–662.

Netzer, C., Klein, C., Kohlhase, J., & Kubisch, C. (2009). New challenges for informed consent through whole genome array testing. *Journal of Medical Genetics, 46*(7), 495–496.

Sharp, M. E., Marder, K. S., Côte, L., Clark, L. N., Nichols, W. C., Vonsattel, J. P., & Alcalay, R. N. (2013). Parkinson's disease with Lewy bodies associated with a heterozygous PARKIN dosage mutation. *Movement Disorders, 29*, 566–568.

Index

Abetalipoproteinaemia, 66
Action myoclonus-renal failure syndrome, 81
Alpha-galactosidase deficiency, 80
L-Arginine, 73–74
Aripiprazole, 29t
ARSACS, 50, 52
Ataxia with vitamin E deficiency, 66
ATXN1, 51t, 57t
ATXN2, 51t, 57t
ATXN3, 51t, 57t
ATXN7, 51t, 57t
Atypical neuroaxonal dystrophy (NAD), 159
Autosomal dominant cerebellar ataxia
    (ADCA), 49–53, 51t, 55–58, 57t, 81.
    see also prion diseases; spinocerebellar
    ataxia
Autosomal dominant hereditary motor
    and sensory neuropathy (HMSN). *see*
    Charcot-Marie-Tooth Disease
Autosomal recessive ataxia of
    Charlevoix-Saguenay. *see* ARSACS

Baclofen, 5, 141
Becker muscular dystrophy, 123–26
Benign familial infantile seizures (BFIS),
    18, 19t, 20, 22
Benign hereditary chorea (BHC), 14
Beta-propeller protein-associated
    neurodegeneration (BPAN), 155–60
Biotin-responsive encephalopathy, 81
Botulinum toxin, 5, 141

CACNA1A, 51t, 57t
Celiac disease, 81
Charcot-Marie-Tooth Disease
    case study, 101
    diagnosis, 102–5
    EGR2, 104
    LITAF, 104
    NEFL, 104
    overview, 102–3
    P0, 104
    PMP22, 103–4, 110–11

treatment, 104
    type 1A, 101–5, 110
Cherry red spot-myoclonus syndrome. *see*
    sialidosis
Cherry red spots, 60, 60f, 61
CHMP2B, 151–55
Chromosome 9 open reading frame 72
    (C9ORF72), 28, 149–53
Chromosome 4 repeat array deletions
    (D4Z4), 129–30
CMT. *see* Charcot-Marie-Tooth Disease
CNBP/ZNF9, 120–21
Coenzyme Q_{10} (CoQ_{10}), 73–74
COL1A2, 12–13, 13f
Co-occurence of Monogenic Disorders,
    163–165
C9orf72. see chromosome 9 open reading
    frame 72 (C9ORF72)
C10orf2/PEO1, 86, 88
Creutzfeldt-Jakob disease (CJD), 144–47

Deep brain stimulation, 5, 15–16
Dentatorubral-pallidoluysian atrophy, 28, 81
Direct-to-consumer genetic testing
    (DTCGT), 167–70
DJ-1, 41–44, 42t
DMD, 124–26
DMPK, 120–22
Dopa-responsive dystonia (DRD)
    case study, 7
    diagnosis, 3, 8–9
    family, counseling, 9–10
    family pedigree, 8f
    GCH1, 3, 7–10, 8f
    treatment, 9–10
    Tyrosine Hydroxylase (TH), 9
Duchenne muscular dystrophy, 124–26
Dystrophinopathies, 123–26
DYT1 dystonia. *see* early-onset dystonia

Early-onset dystonia
    case study, 1
    diagnosis, 2–5, 2f

Early-onset dystonia (*Cont.*)
  DYT6, 3
  DYT25, 3
  family, counseling, 4
  family pedigree, 2*f*
  GCH1, 3, 7–10, 8*f*
  GNAL, 3
  prognosis, 5
  THAP1, 3
  TorsinA (Tor1A), 2–5, 2*f*
  treatment, 4–5
EGR2, 104
Epsilon sarcoglycan (SGCE), 12–15, 13*f*
Eye-of-the-tiger sign, 157, 158*f*

Facioscapulohumeral dystrophy (FSHD),
    127–30
Fatty acid hydroxylase-associated
    neurodegeneration (FAHN), 160
Freidreich ataxa
  cardiomyopathy, 65
  case study, 63, 163
  diagnosis, 64–66, 64*f,* 164
  disease course, 67
  frataxin (FXN), 65–66, 68, 164
  pes cavus, 64, 64*f,* 68
  prevalence, 64, 67
  scoliosis, 63–64, 64*f,* 67–68
  treatment, 65, 67
Frontotemporal dementia (FTD), 133–38,
    149–53
Frontotemporal dementia-amyotrophic
    lateral sclerosis (FTD-ALS), 137,
    149–53, 151*f*
FTL, 160
FUS, 151–52

Gaucher disease
  case study, 45
  diagnosis, 46–47
  GBA, 46–47
  parkinsonism relationship to, 47
  types, 46
GCHI. see early-onset dystonia
Genetic testing
  direct-to-consumer, 167–70
  incidental findings in, 171–74

Gerstmann-Sträussler-Scheinker syndrome
    (GSS), 143–48
GM2 gangliosidosis, 81
GNAL, 3
GRN, 151–52

Harding disease, 97–100
Hereditary neuropathy with liability to
    pressure palsies (HNPP)
  case study, 107
  diagnosis, 108–10
  nerve conduction study, 108–11, 109*f*
  neuropathological findings, 110
  PMP22, 103–4, 110–11
  treatment, 110–11
Hereditary spastic paraplegia (HSP), 139–42
HNPP. *see* hereditary neuropathy with
    liability to pressure palsies
Huntington Disease (HD)
  case study, 25
  diagnosis, 26–28
  family history, 26
  huntingtin, 27–28, 30
  junctophilin-3, 28
  juvenile HD (Westphal variant), 27–28,
    28*f*
  prevalence, 26
  treatment, 29–30, 29*t*

Idebenone, 73, 74, 99, 100
Incidental Findings in Genetic Testing,
    171–174
Inclusion Body Myopathy with
    Paget Disease of Bone and/or
    Frontotemporal Dementia (IBMPFD),
    133–138
Infantile convulsions and choreoathetosis
    (ICCA) syndrome, 18–20
Infantile neuroaxonal dystrophy (INAD), 159

Junctophilin-3, 28

Kearns-Sayre syndrome, 86, 88
KRIT1, 12–13
Kufor Rakeb syndrome, 42*t*
Kuru, 144–45

Lafora body disease, 79
Leber hereditary optic neuropathy (LHON)
   case study, 97
   diagnosis, 98–99
   Harding disease, 97–99, 100
   treatment, 99, 100
Legius syndrome, 115–16
LITAF, 104
LRRK2, 33–37, 168

Machado-Joseph disease, 51*t*, 57*t*
MAPT, 151–52
MECP2, 158, 160
MERRF. *see* myoclonus epilepsy with
   ragged red fibers
Mitochondrial Encephalomyopathy, Lactic
   Acidosis, and Stroke-like episodes
   (MELAS) syndrome
   case study, 69–70
   diagnosis, 72–74
   MRI findings, 71–72, 72*f*, 74
   MT-TL1, 72–74
   muscle biopsy, 71*f*, 73
   treatment, 73, 74
Mitochondrial membrane protein-associated
   neurodegeneration (MPAN), 157–58
Mitochondrial neurogastrointestinal
   encephalopathy syndrome (MNGIE)
   syndrome
   case study, 89–90
   diagnosis, 91–93
   family pedigree, 92*f*
   nerve conduction studies, 91*t*
   prognosis, 94
   thymidine phosphorylase (TYMP), 86–88,
     91–94
   treatment, 93–94
MLPA. *see* multiplex ligation-dependent
   analysis (MLPA)
MT-TL1, 72–74
Myoclonus-dystonia
   case study, 11
   COL1A2, 12–13, 13*f*
   deep brain stimulation, 15–16
   diagnosis, 12–15
   epsilon sarcoglycan (SGCE), 12–15
   family, counseling, 14–15

family pedigree, 13*f*
KRIT1, 12–13
   multiplex ligation-dependent analysis
     (MLPA), 14
   psychiatric features, 12, 15
   treatment, 15–16
Myoclonus epilepsy with ragged red fibers
   (MERRF)
   case study, 77
   diagnosis, 78–82
   muscle biopsy, 80*f*
   prognosis, 82
   surface poly-electromyography (sEMG)
     findings, 78, 78*f*
   treatment, 82
Myotonic dystrophy, 119–21, 163–164

NAD (atypical neuroaxonal dystrophy),
   159
NBAI. *see* neurodegeneration with brain
   iron accumulation
NEFL, 104
NEU1, 60–61
Neuroaxonal dystrophy, 81
Neurodegeneration with brain iron
   accumulation (NBAI)
   atypical neuroaxonal dystrophy (NAD),
     159
   beta-propeller protein-associated
     neurodegeneration (BPAN), 157–61
   case study, 155
   diagnosis, 156–60
   fatty acid hydroxylase-associated
     neurodegeneration (FAHN), 160
   idiopathic, 159–60
   infantile neuroaxonal dystrophy (INAD),
     159
   mitochondrial membrane
     protein-associated neurodegeneration
     (MPAN), 157–58
   MRI findings, 156, 156*f*, 158*f*
   neuroferritinopathy, 160
   pantothenate kinase associated
     neurodegeneration (PKAN), 81, 157,
     158*f*
Neurofibromatosis type I
   case study, 113

diagnosis, 114–17
Legius syndrome, 115–16
NF1, 114– 117
plexiform, 114–15
Neurofibromatosis type I (*Cont.*)
spinal nerve root, 114–15, 117
SPRED1, 116
Neuronal ceroid lipofuscinosis, 79
NF1, 114–17
Niemann-Pick type C, 156
Noonan syndrome, 116

Olanzapine, 29*t*
OPA1, 86–88
Oppenheim dystonia. *see* early-onset dystonia

P0, 104
Pantothenate kinase associated
neurodegeneration (PKAN), 81, 157,
158*f*, 160
Paraplegin, 141
Parkin, 39–44, 171–74
Parkinson disease (dominant)
alpha-synuclein (SNCA), 35, 36*t*, 37
case study, 33
diagnosis, 34–35, 36*f*
direct-to-consumer genetic testing, 167–70
family, counseling, 35–36
family pedigree, 35*f*
forms of, 36*t*
LRRK2, 33–37, 168
treatment, 36
VPS35, 35, 36*t*, 37
Parkinson disease (recessive)
case study, 39
diagnosis, 40–42, 44
DJ-1, 41–44, 42*t*
family, counseling, 42–43
family pedigree, 41*f*
forms of, 42*t*
Kufor Rakeb syndrome, 42*t*
multiplex ligation-dependent analysis
(MLPA), 41–42, 172
Parkin, 40–44, 41*f*, 42*t*, 171–74
PINK1, 41–44, 42*t*
treatment, 43
Paroxysmal dyskinesia

case study, 17
diagnosis, 18–22
*proline-rich transmembrane protein 2
(PRRT2)*, 18, 22
treatment, 18–22
types, 19*t*
Paroxysmal exertion-induced dyskinesia
(PED), 18, 19*t*, 20
Paroxysmal nonkinesigenic dyskinesias
(PNKD), 18, 19*t*, 20
Pimozide, 29*t*
PINK1, 41–44, 42*t*
Piracetam, 82
PLA2G6, 159
PMP22, 103–4, 110–11
POLG-related mitochondrial disease
case study, 85
diagnosis, 86–88
POLG, 86–88
treatment, 87
Poly-hill sign, 128
Prion diseases, 28, 143–48
Prion protein (PRNP), 28, 144, 145, 146*f*,
147
Prion protein (PrP), 145
Progressive external ophthalmoplegia
(PEO), 86–88, 141–42
*Proline-rich transmembrane protein 2
(PRRT2)*, 18–22
Proximal myotonic myopathy (PROMM),
119–21

Refsum disease, 66
Rett syndrome, 158–60

SENDA. *see* static encephalopathy with
neurodegeneration in adulthood
SGCE (epsilon sarcoglycan). *see* epsilon
sarcoglycan (SGCE)
Sialidosis
case study, 59
cherry red spots, 60, 60*f*, 61
diagnosis, 60–61
family pedigree, 61*f*
infantile, 60, 61
NEU1, 60–61
SLC25A4, 86, 88

SNCA, 35, 36*t*, 37
SPAST, 140, 142
Spastic-ataxia phenotype, 49–53, 55–58, 140, 140*f*
SPG7. *see* hereditary spastic paraplegias with signs of ataxia
Spinocerebellar ataxia type 2
  case study, 49
  diagnosis, 50–53
  MRI findings, 50, 51*f*
Spinocerebellar ataxia type 17
  case study, 55
  diagnosis, 28, 56–58
  Huntington disease phenocopy syndrome, 28, 56–58
SPRED1, 116
Static encephalopathy with neurodegeneration in adulthood (SENDA), 155–61
Steinert disease, 120–21
Sulpiride, 29*t*

TBP, 57*t*
Tetrabenazine, 29*t*
THAP1, 3
Thymidine phosphorylase (TYMP), 86–88, 91–94
Tiapride, 29*t*
TorsinA (Tor1A), 2–5, 2*f*
Trihexiphenidyl, 4–5
Tyrosine Hydroxylase (TH), 9

Unverricht-Lundborg disease, 79–80

Valosin-containing protein (VCP), 135–36, 151–52
Von Recklinghausen disease. *see* neurofibromatosis type I
VPS35, 35, 36*t*, 37

WDR45, 158–60
Whipple disease, 81
Writer's cramp, 12